ESSENTIAL OILS FOR BEGINNERS

Discover This Guide About How to Effectively Use
Essential Oils

(The Complete Guide to Losing Weight Fast Using
Essential Oils)

Melba Crispin

Published By Andrew Zen

Melba Crispin

All Rights Reserved

Essential Oils for Beginners: Discover This Guide About How to Effectively Use Essential Oils (The Complete Guide to Losing Weight Fast Using Essential Oils)

ISBN 978-1-77485-245-3

Legal & Disclaimer

The information contained in this book is not designed to replace or take the place of any form of medicine or professional medical advice. The information in this book has been provided for educational and entertainment purposes only.

The information contained in this book has been compiled from sources deemed reliable, and it is accurate to the best of the Author's knowledge; however, the Author cannot guarantee its accuracy and validity and cannot be held liable for any errors or omissions. Changes are periodically made to this book. You must consult your doctor or get professional medical advice before using any of the suggested remedies, techniques, or information in this book.

Upon using the information contained in this book, you agree to hold harmless the Author from and against any damages, costs, and expenses, including any legal fees potentially resulting from the application of any of the information provided by this guide. This disclaimer applies to any damages or injury caused by the use and application, whether directly or indirectly, of any advice or information presented, whether for breach of contract, tort, negligence, personal injury, criminal intent, or under any other cause of action.

You agree to accept all risks of using the information presented inside this book. You need to consult a professional medical practitioner in order to ensure you are both able and healthy enough to participate in this program.

TABLE OF CONTENTS

INTRODUCTION.. 1

CHAPTER 1: ESSENTIAL OILS FOR BEGINNERS.................... 3

CHAPTER 2: UTILIZE ESSENTIAL OIL 9

CHAPTER 3: CHEATS SPRAY 18

CHAPTER 4: ESSENTIAL OILS FOR NERVE PAIN................. 34

CHAPTER 5: THINGS TO TAKE INTO ACCOUNT WHEN
PURCHASING ESSENTIAL OILS 44

CHAPTER 6: THE WAY TO GET THE HEALTH BENEFITS OF
ESSENTIAL OILS 53

CHAPTER 7: COMMONLY ASKED QUESTIONS 57

CHAPTER 8: CHOOSING THE ESSENTIAL OIL THAT'S RIGHT
FOR YOU 78

CHAPTER 9: DEPRESSION AND ANXIETY ESSENTIAL OIL
RECIPES 83

CHAPTER 10: HOLISTIC USES.. 87

CHAPTER 11: THE PRECAUTIONS TO BE AWARE OF PRIOR
TO USING ESSENTIAL OILS... 98

CHAPTER 12: WHAT'S THAT? A GUIDE TO ESSENTIAL OILS

.... **102**

CHAPTER 13: LAVENDER ESSENTIAL OIL 107

CHAPTER 14: HEALTH AND WELLNESS........................... 131

CHAPTER 15: ESSENTIAL OILS FOR MENTAL HEALTH 136

CHAPTER 16: ESSENTIAL OIL RECIPES FOR RELAXATION

AND STRESS RELIEVEMENT... 140

CHAPTER 17: WHAT TO FIND THE BEST ESSENTIAL OILS 158

CHAPTER 18: EXTRACTION OF ESSENTIAL OILS.............. 164

CHAPTER 19: AROMATHERAPY HEALTH BENEFITS OF

AROMATHERAPY... 171

CONCLUSION... 182

Introduction

You're tired of the pills with side effects, and need something that is natural and more holistic. The internet has been a source of confusion, because there's website after site with suggestions and tips for managing discomfort with essential oils and aromatherapy and you're left in doubt about which ones actually work. You've attempted to read numerous books about aromatherapy, but the terms used in clinical practice have caused you to scratch your head. This book contains everything you need to begin managing your pain naturally with essential oils in an easy-to-follow layout.

I've gathered my years of experience and research in bringing you an aromatherapy guide that takes the guesswork out making essential oil blends. The book includes information, essential oil profiles and recipes for blends of essential oils to start your journey. The only remaining question is:

What are you putting off?

Chapter 1: Essential Oils For Beginners

Are you new to the idea of using essential oils? It is important to know several important bits of information you have to understand before you start. This will allow you to not only apply the essential oils in a more effective manner, but also give you knowledge which will enable you to go one step further. In the end, there are a lot of things you can accomplish using these oils.

For you to get to where you want to be, here are a few of the basics that any beginner must be aware of about essential oils:

They aren't really oils. They don't contain the fats that typically make up the oil-based products. But, they are a extremely concentrated plant constituents that also has potent cosmetic as well as medicinal properties. Many consider them to be the vitality of the plant which is a sign of how potent it could be.

The majority of essential oils possess powerful antibacterial, antifungal and antiviral effects. This means that, in addition to the typical uses for them medical and cosmetic are also a good option to add these oils to your cleaning products. The best part? It's 100% natural and doesn't emit toxic fumes that are harmful to your health and that of your family members. The most effective ones to do this are lemon, peppermint and rosemary.

Essential oils are small when you look at them molecularly. This means they can be readily absorbed by your skin, which means that their effects will be absorbed much faster and perform more efficiently. If you want to heal and nourish your skin, essential oils are your best choice. But it should be noted that, unlike other products for beauty essential oils don't build up or leave residues on the body, even after long periods of usage. After they've delivered the beneficial substances, they are absorbed and out of your body.

Essential oils of rosemary will help you to study more effectively. Recent studies have proven that smelling it will assist you in keeping more information, and at the same time improve your memory recall , which can improve your results when it comes to tests. This can be attributed to the smell that produces relaxing effects.

Fragrance oils aren't the same. Fragrance oils are most of the time produced synthetically even though they claim to be "natural scent". Essential oils however are made from plants which is organic.

Essential oils can't be patentable because they are entirely natural. That means you won't ever find any in a drug. Most mainstream medical professionals don't endorse or suggest the use of it as a viable alternative to synthetic drugs. Drug companies will not spend their time studying them since they claim there is no revenue to be earned out of these substances. The truth is that our understanding about essential oils as well as their applications is extremely restricted. What we know is based on information which has been handed through the ages of ancient medicine and personal experience and experimentation.

It takes a lot of plants to create essential oils. This is the reason they are quite costly when you're shopping for the best quality. In order to produce a pound of essential oil it takes the equivalent of 4000 pounds Bulgarian roses must be processed. Certain varieties require less, for example, lavenders, which require just 100 pounds of plants to make one pounds of oil. This process leaves the oil extremely concentrated and therefore extremely powerful.

Many essential oils aren't meant to be used in a pure form to apply on the skin.

Instead, it is recommended to mix them with butters, carrier oils waxes, and other diluting methods you would like to use. This is due to the fact that they're so concentrated that using them alone could cause an uncomfortable skin reaction. Also, be aware the possibility of having any allergies.

Importantly, be aware of the following warnings:

Do you want to find out whether you're allergic to a specific type in essential oils? Here's how you can test. Take a drop of oil with half a tablespoon of the carrier oil, and rub it on the upper part of the arm just to the inside in the area where the sensitive skin is. Let it sit for about two hours. If there is no redness or itchiness appears, then you're not sensitized to the essential oil.

Do not consume essential oils, particularly the wintergreen and eucalyptus. Although there are some which can be utilized in toothpaste, it must be thoroughly diluted to be certain that it's safe for consumption. In reality, you should be aware of kinds that are so poisonous that even contact with the skin is not recommended. Be assured because these are the most rare and they aren't readily available in shops.

Chapter 2: Utilize Essential Oil

The body requires all essential oils. However, this does not mean that you should take any amount of the oil. It is important to keep in mind this: these oil are corrosive and can cause an enormous harm to your body. This chapter can help you figure out the most effective method of ensuring that you're consuming essential oils required for your body to function at a high level.

Inhaling the Oil

It is among the easiest ways to consume essential oils. When you inhale essential oil, you're increasing your senses as well as stimulating the reaction you want to receive from the body. There are a variety of techniques are required to use when breathing essential oils.

Direct Inhaling

The best way to inhale is to inhale directly. You can sniff the oil to make sure that you've got the content you want from the oil.

Diffusion

The other method you can use to take in the oil is to do so through diffusion. In this way the oil is transformed into the form of vapor, suspended in air. Make sure to choose the diffuser in a way that does not cause heat to the contents since this can alter the nature of the nutrients the oil is a source of.

Make use of a humidifier

Another method you can employ is humidification. Purchase a humidifier and start to warm the water. Grab a tissue and put a few drops essential oil onto it. Be sure to making sure that you do not put the oil directly into the humidifier as the oil will rise up to the top, making the vapor ineffective to breathe. Instead, put the tissue over the steam that is coming out of.

Steam

Make a large vessel with water. Add a few drops oil to the water. place your head over your nose while taking in the aroma. It is important to breathe in slowly and deeply to feel the rhythm.

The application of the oil on Certain Body Parts

It is essential to make sure that the oil you require is applied and rubbed as per the instructions on the side of the container. It is necessary be able to reduce the amount of oil by using vegetable oileither refined or pure oil. It is recommended to do this in accordance with the chart you have been given. This chart can help you limit the damage can be caused for your skin. There are certain areas that where you can apply the essential oil to.

The forehead

The temples behind your ears

The neck

The Crown of the Head

The the soles of your feet

The upper part of your ankle

There are a variety of techniques are required to adhere to when taking in essential oils. This article outlines the most basic and simple techniques you can effectively apply.

Direct Application

This is the most straightforward method to apply oil to the skin that is on the body. You can apply just a few drops and apply it to the area for two to three minutes.

Massage Oil

Another method to make sure your body is absorbing the oil is by the massage. Drop three to three drops into your palm and then rub your palms together in circular motion. If you're directly applying the oil to your skin, then you need to apply some pressure on the skin. In this way, you'll be able to make sure that the oil you apply isn't likely to cause any type of irritation to your skin. Be aware the fact that oils with essential components are extremely powerful and can cause severe inflammation to the skin.

If you are finding that it's hard get your hands rub the oil in a gentle manner without getting an irritation, add a teaspoon of oil from a vegetable to every essential oil to even out the power.

Internal Consumption

This is the most effective approach to go about it since it will not cause any harm to the general health of your body. It is, however, risky to consume it internally because essential oils are powerful and can influence the body. This section will assist you in understanding the best way to ensure the amount of essential oil doesn't harm the body.

Research was conducted. The results of this research show that there are essential oils that work better when taken orally. Only the purest version that these oils are in has been confirmed to be safe to consume orally. They are commonly utilized as supplements to diets. The amount of oil to be diluted depends on the age of the individual. The health status of the individual is crucial. Learn the directions for each product before administering oil orally.

Make a capsule and make sure to fill it with your essential oil. Make sure you rinse it off with plenty of water.

When you drink milk or water throughout the day, it is possible to add a few drops this essential oil. for instance 1 or 2 drops.

If you're making the bread, or making food preparations be sure you include a few drops of the oil to your food items.

Drop it on your tongue and then swallow it immediately. It is important to be very cautious in this process as essential oils are very powerful. You must examine the oil using the methods above before putting the oil directly onto your tongue.

Responsible use of essential oils

Essential oils pose a risk to use for general. You must be able to manage yourself and the oil in case you intend to apply them to your body. This section will cover the fundamental techniques you'll be required to consider when the use of essential oils.

Utilize a drop-orifice. This will help you make sure that you're adhering to the proper dosage as recommended by your doctor or other health experts. In the event that you are using an opening that reduces the amount of drop, you'll be able to make sure that your children or any other child won't be able consume the oil. They will be given essential oil at times whenever it is needed. If you discover that your child has consumed more food, you'll need consult a physician. Before that, however you should provide your child with milk.

If you have children in your home, it's ideal to speak with an experienced health professional prior to deciding whether you want to give your child any essential oils.

If you plan to try new essential oils, try them on a small patch on your face. You can test it on any surface because the sensitivity varies. If your skin is turning bright red or is becoming hot, you'll need to cleanse it right away. It is likely that the water you use is less effective.

Try to experiment with a new oil at each time. You can make a blend of oils if that's what you want to do. Place a few drops on your body, and wait for a couple of minutes. If your skin doesn't exhibit any negative reactions, you are able to continue using the oil.

Certain essential oils that could cause irritation to your eyes. They can cause irritation to sensitive parts on your body. If you've used essential oils and then begin to contact your lenses, you could cause damage to them for a long time, thereby damaging your eyes. If you discover that this happened by accident you should apply 1 - 2 drops vegetable oil to your eyes right away.

Do not put essential oils in your ears!

If you're using the pure oils of citrus, you could discover that exposure to sunlight has various impacts on the skin.

Do not apply essential oils to your skin areas where you've used cosmetics. The cosmetics could absorb essential oils deep into the body. The oil could then be found in your fat tissue, in the bloodstream, or even your skin.

Never apply essential oils to the skin that is damaged or affected due to chemical burns.

Chapter 3: Cheats Spray

The aroma of this oil is like Christmas. I love the Cheats splash essential oil formula and would love to give it to my friends and family. It's very easy to use and I have it in my house and in my diaper bag to take on trips.

It is possible to use it for:

Toys for children that are clean

Clean public restrooms

Wipe off cutting boards

Cleanse leafy foods

Freshen gym bags

Clean up the plane's armrests and serving plates

Spray around the room to rid it of unpleasant odors

The benefits that this spray can serve are endless. Additionally, it's incredibly simple to create.

What you'll require:

2 oz. Dark glass splash bottle

1 teaspoon witch hazel common

10-15 drops of Cheats for Youthful Living oil

Almost 2 oz. of refined water

Instructions:

To make the perfect splash bottle Add 10 to 15 drops of Cheats oil. Then , add 1 teaspoon of witch hazel. Fill the bottle up with distilled water. . It's that simple! This is among my most-loved DIY essential oil formulas!

Glossy Hair Serum

Who doesn't want beautiful gorgeous, stunning hair? In the case of stress, blues from babies or aging, our hair may begin to lose its shape, crack or dull in its shine. I really enjoy using this DIY essential oil recipe to improve my hair's appears and smells.

You'll need:

2 ounce dark glass dropper bottle

About 2 ounces castor oil

10 drops essential rosemary oil

Five drops of lavender are essential oil

5 drops of ylang-premier oil

Instructions:

Pour 2 oz. of Castor Oil into your dropper bottle. Add the other oils. Cover the dropper with a cover and shake the bottle. Massage the mixture into your hair each morning. It should be left for at least 20 minutes before washing. You can apply it before going to going to bed! If the serum is too oily, you can replace the castor oil by adding 2 8 oz. of refined water and one teaspoon witch hazel.

All Abstentions Salve

This is an excellent multi-purpose ointment, which is perfect for the skin. Lemon and Melaleuca provide numerous benefits which include antibacterial. Lavender oil is a relaxing one well-known for its effects on the skin. I really enjoy carrying this ointment around in my bag. It can also be used as a hand moisturizing product in the winter months when it is cold and wet.

What you'll require:

1 ounce glass moisturizer container

5 drops of lemon oil

5 drops of lavender oil

Five drops of tea tree (melaleuca alternifolia) oil

About 2 8 oz. of coconut oil that has not been cooked

Instructions:

Scoop 2 oz. of coconut oil uncooked into a glass dish. Pour the oil in. Stir the mixture well with the steel spoon or fork. Scoop the mixture into a glass container for cream and place the cover on. Store in a cool, dark place. Apply directly on skin as required. This is a wonderful one for mothers!

Cozy Exfoliation Body Scrub

Does it make sense to say that the skin is our largest organ? To care for it in a proper manner, we need to be taking care to remove dead skin cells each day. The process of skin brushing is an excellent method to do this, particularly when you pair it with a regular body scrub. This luxurious peeling scrub will leave your skin a stunning shine!

What you'll require:

8 ounce glass container

White covers - not mandatory for an exclusive appearance

4 oz. of olive oil uncooked

8 oz. of sea salt

5 drops of frankincense, lavender and ylang

Instructions:

Make sure you measure your salt, then empty it directly into the dish of a large glass. Add olive oil and mix thoroughly using a metallic spoon. Add your essential oils and blend your mix. Scoop the mixture into the glass container. Secure it with a white cover. Mark. Store in a cool, dark place. Scoop out a silver buck's worth of scour. Apply it to your the body prior to showering. Repeat every week. Your skin will be grateful.

The Exfoliation Facial Scrub is expensive and costly.

The recipe is similar to the one as above, but we're using sugar in place of salt due to the fact that it's more gentle and healthier for your skin. There are three combinations of oils that will suit your skin type.

You'll need:

8 glass containers of 8 ounces

White lids are not required but can give your home a distinctive style

Half cup olive oil raw

1 cup raw sugar

For normal skin 5 drops Each of Lavender, Frankincense and ylang

For oily skin 5 drops of oil extracted from the carrot seed and tea tree oils, and Frankincense

For older or dry skin 5 drops of each of patchouli, geranium oil , and the frankincense

To make a special treat 5 drops each of jasmine, rose and sacred oils of frankincense

Instructions:

Measure the sugar you want to use and pour it into the large glass bowl. Add olive oil, and mix well using an iron spoon. Include your essential oils and continue stirring the mixture. Scoop the mixture slowly into the glass container. Cover tightly with a lid of white and the label. Place in a dark area =. Scoop out the equivalent of a silver dollar's worth of scrub and apply it weekly.

Muscle Love Bath Salts

These salts are ideal for people who want to relax their muscles after intense exercise or gardening.

What you'll require:

Glass container of eight ounces

White lids are not required however it gives an interesting look

10 drops panaway and/or aroma siez

5 drops copiaba

1 cup of Epsom salts

Instructions:

Make sure you put your Epsom salts in an enormous glass bowl. Add the essential oils and mix well using an iron spoon. Pour the mixture into an 8 ounce glass bottle and secure with lid. Scoop about 1/4-1/2 cup and then place it in an ice bath as needed. Your athlete will be happy!

Coffee Cellulite Scrub

It is the most original of my DIY essential oil recipes for essential oils. Coffee is known as a stimulant, and it can help our body with breaking down fat that are stored beneath the skin. The grapefruit as well as Cypress oils are both high-quality lymph nodes boosters. When combined, this makes an ideal scrub!

You'll need:

8 glass containers with a glass lid

White lids are not required You can choose the color you prefer.

Ten drops grapefruit oils

5 drops of oil from cypress

1 cup natural espresso

Half an olive oil cup

Instructions:

Measure your coffee , then pour into an enormous glass bowl. Add olive oil to the bowl and mix well using the help of a spoon made of metal. Incorporate the oils and stir the mixture. Scoop the mixture slowly into the glass container. Seal tightly and label. Store in a cool, dark location. Scoop up a silver dollar's worth amount of scrub and apply all over your body before you shower.

Balancing Fragrance Combination

People with a keen nose will enjoy this fragrance blend. I've gifted this to family members as well as friends numerous times. The blend of oils makes people feel happy and healthy. The oils listed are safe for babies as well as pregnant mothers and breastfeeding mothers.

What you'll require:

1 darkish glass roll-on bottle

1TB coconut oil extracted

Three drops of grapefruit oils

2 drops of Grankincense oil

A drop or two of oil from copiaba

One drop Bergamot Oil

Instructions:

The oil drops should be added to the roll-on bottle. The remaining portion of the roll-on bottle with a light carrier oil like coconut oil that has been extracted. Seal the bottle tightly. Keep in an area that is cool and dark. Sprinkle on pulse points as needed.

Refreshing Cologne

Who says essential oils are just for women? Give your guy an oil for men that can help improve his health and let him smell amazing. Balsam Fir is a great scent that is reminiscent of the Christmas tree, while Cedar-wood has an aroma of musk that's perfect for the man you love.

You'll need:

1 dark glass roll-on bottle

1 TB of coconut oil abstracted

3 drops Balsam oil from Fir

Three drops Cedar wood oil

Instructions:

Make sure to add your oil drops to the roll-on bottle. Fill the remainder of your roll-on container with a light carrier oil like coconut oil extracted. Securely cover the bottle. Place in a dark area. Apply pulse points to the areas when needed.

Fresh and Minty Shaving Cream

Are you aware that the most shaving creams for men contain strong chemicals and perfumes? I love this homemade blend that makes the skin feel amazing, thanks to the coconut and shea oil and also energized due to the peppermint oil.

It is possible to add any essential oil that you'd like to alter the smell.

What you'll require:

8 glass containers with a glass lid

White lids are optional. it's up to you personal taste

1/3 cup shea butter

1/3 cup coconut oil

3 TB of olive oil that is uncooked

1 teaspoon castile soap

7 drops of oil containing peppermint

Instructions:

Add your shea spread as well as coconut oil into a twofold burner. Place the burner on low heat and allow the fats to melt. Take them off the burner and transfer the oil to the tumbler dish. Add your olive oil. Let cool before adding to your Castile soap along with essential oils. Place in the fridge for about up to 60 mins or till the mix has hardened. After that, take it out from fridge and blend the mixture using a blender until you create a whipped cream-like composition. Scoop into your glass container. Seal it tightly and keep in a dark, cool location. Scoop out a silver-buck's worth of cream and apply it before shaving.

Eliminating Shaving Gel

Men prefer an oil-based gel instead of creams, and that's why I came up with this blend to help them use. Aloe vera is"the "gel" and gives your skin a smooth. Lemongrass and Grapefruit scents are divine and help to increase blood flow and allow the lymphatic system to function!

You'll need:

eight ounce dim glass pump bottle

3/4 cup aloe vera gel

1/4 cup olive oil

7 drops of oil from lemongrass

Seven drops grapefruit oils

Instructions:

Utilizing funnels using a funnel, pour the aloe gel into the glass. Include the olive oil as well as your other essential oils. Secure the bottle by closing an open pump and vigorously shake. Keep it in a cool, dark area. When needed, apply it to the skin prior to shaving.

Inspiring After Shave

This is the top picks from the DIY essential oil formulations due to the fact that Orange + Sandalwood is Heaven! Each of these oil-based remedies are perfect for this ointment for the face, and not just due to the smell, but also because they moisturize the skin.

You'll need:

8 Ounce dark glass pump bottle

1/2 cup aloe vera gel

Half cup of witch hazel

2 TB jojoba oil

1 teaspoon vitamin E oil

10 drops of orange oil

10 drops of sandalwood oil

Instructions:

Utilizing a funnel, pour the gel of aloe vera into the container. Add your witch-hazel, Jojoba, and Vitamin E oils. Then add the other ingredients. Close your container with the top of your pump, and shake thoroughly. Place it in a cool dark location. When needed, apply it on the face after shaving.

Chapter 4: Essential Oils For Nerve Pain

Nerve pain can manifest various ways. It could also be an offshoot from other ailments, like diabetes or carpal tunnel. It can be anything from numbness, tingling and pain in the tips of fingers to sharp painful pains on the bottoms the feet, or a sciatic nerve that shoots pain across one leg. It's not a pleasant experience and there's no solution to fix the damage after it's happened. But there's an option to control the issue and keep it manageable. Here's a list essential oils that you'll require:

(Note that I've included the Latin name since common names are interchangeable.)

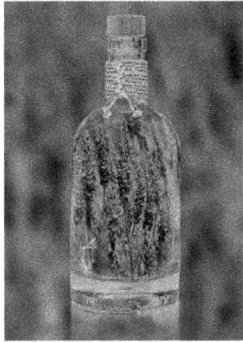

Chamomile, German

(Matricaria recutica) The essential oil (Matricaria recutica) is renowned for its spasm relief properties and reducing pain. It is among the most commonly used essential oils used to manage pain.

Chamomile, Roman

(Chamamelum nobile) (Chamamelum nobile) that same class as above shares the same characteristics. It also functions as an sedative for nerves.

Clove

(Syzygium aromaticum) (Syzygium aromaticum) is one of the most well-known essential oils that aid in relief from pain and pain management. It is possible to apply the clove powder that you cook on abscesses and it will ease the burden of the discomfort. Since it is an essential oil it is able to be applied to more places to gain more benefits. It is recommended to use it in small quantities only.

Eucalyptus

(Eucalyptus globeulus) It's true that this essential oil is not just used with respiratory problems as well as with neuralgia cases.

Geranium

(Pelaronium graveolens) The oil has been used to treat neuralgia.

Helichrysum

(Helichrysum angustifolium) The essential oil contains properties that can treat neuralgia. This oil can trigger breakouts in those who are hypersensitive.

True Lavender

(Lavandula angustifolia) (Lavandula angustifolia) the most commonly used essential oils and is available in the market. It is a good option for sciatic nerve pain.

Peppermint

(Mentha piperita) It aids in cases of neuralgia or pain spasms. There are many more applications that are described in the other chapters.

All Purpose Nerve Pain Oil

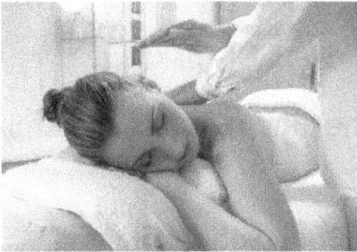

4 8 ounces Sweet Almond or Apricot Kernel oil

1/5 tsp Peppermint EO

1/5 teaspoon German Chamomile EO

15 Drops True Lavender EO

5 drops of Clove 5 drops of Clove

All the components thoroughly and apply the mixture to the areas that are affected.

Before bed Massage oil

4 pounds Sweet Almond or Apricot Kernel oil

1/5 tsp of Roman Chamomile EO

1/5 teaspoon Eucalyptus EO

15 Drops of Geranium EO

5 Drops Clove 5 Drops Clove

Follow the instructions on mixing and using.

Neuralgia Body Soak

1 Cup Epsom Salts

12 Cup Sea salt

1/4 Cup baking Soda

1/4 Cup Borax (It's a natural mineral)

1/5 tsp of Roman Chamomile EO

1/5 tsp of peppermint EO

15 Drops of Geranium Oil

5 Drops Clove 5 Drops Clove

One Ounce Sweet Almond or Apricot Kernel Oil

You use a lesser quantity of the carrier oil since you're also using minerals and salts to dilute essential oils.

Mix the oils, then put aside.

Mix all dry ingredients together and put aside.

Add the oils slowly to the dry ingredients, blending it thoroughly.

* Put in a closed container for the night.

• Add mineral baths in 14 Cup increments into warm water.

Mix well into the bath water. Let it take a bath and.

* You could also pour the mixture in 1/8 cup measure into the bowl of hot water and use it to make compress.

This can ease the neuralgia, as well as your nerves, allowing you to rest better in the night. It also helps with Restless Leg Syndrome.

Neuralgia Body Soak II

1 Cup Epsom Salts

12 Cup Sea salt

1/4 Cup baking Soda

1/4 Cup Borax (It's a natural mineral)

1/5 tsp Helichrysum EO

1/5 tsp peppermint EO

15 Drops of Geranium EO

5 Drops Lavender EO

One Ounce Sweet Almond or Apricot Kernel Oil

You use a lesser volume of oil carrier since you're also using minerals and salts to dilute essential oils.

Mix the oils together and put aside.

Mix dry ingredients together and put aside.

Add the oils slowly to dry ingredients, mixing it thoroughly.

* Put in a sealed container for the night.

• Add mineral baths in 14 Cup increments into warm water.

Mix well with the bath water. Let it take a bath and.

* You can also pour the mix in 1/8 cup measurements into an unheated bowl and use it to make compress.

This can ease the neuralgia and your nerves, which will help you rest better in the night. This can also help to treat Restless Leg Syndrome.

Salve on-the-spot

1 cup Sweet Almond or Apricot Kernel oil

1/8-cup Beeswax Beads

2/5 tsp Peppermint EO

2/5 tsp True Lavender EO

10 drops of Geranium EO

10 drops of Clove 10 Drops of Clove

* In a double boiler add the oil and beeswax.

• Melt the honey.

* Mix essential oils.

* Make sure the salve is warm , but still mixable prior to adding the essential oils to stop the oils from vaporizing.

* Let cool overnight

* Apply the cream to the affected region as required to ease discomfort.

Ointment for quick and dirty cleaning

4 ounces non-petroleum jelly

1/5 teaspoon Eucalyptus EO

1/5 tsp GeraniumEO

15 Drops True Lavender EO

5 Drops Clove 5 Drops Clove

* Heat the jelly gently until it is melted in the double boiler.

* Place the contents in a sealed container that is tightly sealed.

Mix essential oils and add them to the jelly when it is warm

* Allow it to chill overnight.

Apply pressure to the affected area whenever needed to ease the pain.

Chapter 5: Things to Take into Account When Purchasing Essential Oils

Utilizing essential oils is one of the most effective ways to improve your health overall and that of those who are around you. They provide a broad benefit to keeping your health in check as well as your home. They are the most effective items you can buy. To make your experience enjoyable, it is important to focus on the best quality as well as healing properties and scent.

When you are purchasing essential oils, there are some factors to keep in your mind, such as the purpose you intend to utilize the essential oil for and the quality of oil you require and so on. If you are planning to start using certain essential oils to your children, your family and pets, it is suggested to purchase pure therapeutic quality oils. There are many locations where you can purchase essential oils. There are several essential oils and plant varieties brands to pick from.

When choosing an essential oil, it is all about what you want to treat or stop as well as how effective you'd prefer them to be, and the final point is what price you intend to reach your objectives. The price of essential oils is a lot different because some oils are of higher quality than other products. The variables that influence the price of essential oils include where the plant comes from as well as the rarity of the plant as well as controls for quality that are implemented by distillers.

Essential oils of poor quality or oils that are adulterated aren't considered to be therapeutic. This is due to the fact that they could produce harmful side effects or offer no therapeutic benefits. Pure essential oils consist of only the concentrated aromatic compounds that come from the plant, without any alteration. The adulterations and additives which can be added to oils in order to reduce production costs could contain chemical dilutants certain artificial oils, blend of inexpensive oil and costly alcohol, etc.

If you're a professional aromatherapist or just a beginner with essential oils, the quality is a constant factor to consider. There are several aspects that impact the potency of oils, and they are as follows The following are the most important:

The production method.

Methods of harvesting and cultivation.

The portion of the plant which was utilized.

The source of essential oil.

The climate in conditions the plant grown as well as the time of harvest.

How oil is stored and how for how long.

There are a few aspects that one must take into consideration when purchasing essential oils:

Proper packaging, as well as the labeling requirements.

How knowledgeable the founders of the company are.

When you are buying essential oils, make sure you're aware of terms such as "fragrance oil" or words like "nature the same oil" or "perfumes oil" because these terms indicate that the product you're looking at isn't pure or isn't a one essential oil.

The way the plants are grown purchasing essential oils supplied from local sustainably-minded growers more beneficial than buying organic , due to excellent quality because of the personal attention given to local farmers.

It is important to consider the process of distillation used to make the oil since the most effective distillation methods are the ones that change the oil's essential properties in the least amount while with the greatest beneficial properties.

It is also worth considering the cost aspect since to get the best, you need to spend a bit of money.

It is also a matter of the credibility of the business that you purchase your products from be sure it has an excellent reputation in terms of their service and quality, as well as the prices of the essential oils they use.

The therapeutic properties of the oil should be taken into consideration and be aware of the healing properties of the oil.

It is also important to take into consideration the fragrance that the oil has regardless of how effective the benefits are, they're not worth the price. If you don't like the smell, you'll probably not make use of it.

Methods for application of essential oils

Pure essential oils provide many benefits for health and it's crucial to be aware that the method used will affect the result. One thing you should keep in your mind is that nearly every essential oil must be applied without diluting the skin. Essential oils are typically applied in three methods i.e. aromatically or topically, as well as internally.

When you are using essential oils, there are certain signs you must be on the lookout for These are:

The green symbol signifies the safety of using with no diluting as directed.

The orange symbol is required to be moderate dilution in order to be safe.

The red symbol indicates the need for strong dilution and with a precautionary approach.

Application of aromas

The aromatherapy application of essential oils is believed as the one most sought-after. Aromatic uses go beyond simply the concept of having a pleasing scent. We can experience the beneficial properties of essential oils because they are absorbed into the bloodstream through inhalation. Essential aromas are processed in the olfactory system and the limbic system. This can be described as the exact system responsible for our thoughts emotions, feelings and even memories aiding one to relax and feel peaceful.

The scent that one inhale is made up of the same elements that make up its oil. It is possible to inhale essential oils using particular devices, and also by using different methods e.g. diffusers, dry evaporation steam, and spray.

Topically

Applying essential oils topically is simple , however it is delicate. Many essential oils are suitable for use topically. However , there are variations in their use due to the fact that some contain restrictions on frequency or dilution. It is crucial to determine your skin's type since when you suffer from sensitive skin, you must always reduce the amount of oil. If you dilute it, the efficacy of the oil does not decrease and in fact, it helps boost absorption rates by stopping loss of the oil and reduces the possibility of having an allergic reaction to the skin.

Internally

It is important to keep in mind that only a handful of essential oils are safe to use internally , and many people do not use the oils internally as it could cause some adverse impacts on the body. There are certain essential oils considered safe for internal use , however they nevertheless require caution. Things you need to be aware of when taking essential oils internally are described below:

More is less.

Increase frequency prior to the decreases.

Limit your daily doses.

Always dilute.

Some people should stay clear of applying it to themselves.

Chapter 6: The Way to get the health benefits of Essential Oils

Below are some health issues that essential oils may treat

Depression, Stress, and Anxiety

Depression, stress, and anxiety are common among individuals that if they are not treated can lead to a serious ailments. Aromatherapy can go far in tackling this kind of vice. A few studies have demonstrated that the aroma or flavor of certain essential oils may aid in treating stress and anxiety.

But, this research has been unable to prove real and is regarded as a false belief since there isn't any evidence to support the assertions. Therefore, the remedy for stress and anxiety that relies on essential oils' scent or flavor is currently unproven.

Another way to use essential oils to ease stress is to massage your body with the essential oil. The use of essential oils to massage the body parts can help lessen stress, although the effect may only last a few minutes while the massage is performed. But research have been conducted recently and the results show that aromatherapy isn't effective in alleviating anxiety.

Sleep and insomnia

To ensure a restful sleep, especially for women who have just given birth or suffer from heart conditions, inhaling and inhaling the aroma of lavender oil is extremely beneficial for this.

Migraines and Headaches

Studies conducted in the past revealed that when a blend of ethanol and peppermint oil is applied to the forehead of those suffering from headaches, the mix assists in relieving headache. Recent studies confirmed the earlier findings. If peppermint oil combined with lavender oil is applied to the forehead, it can help relieve headaches. A mixture of sesame oil and chamomile can be effective in the treatment of headaches as well as migraines.

Reducing Inflammation

Research has proven that essential oils have anti-inflammatory properties within nature i.e. they are able to help combat inflammation. But, the efficacy of this study hasn't been proven on people who suffer from inflammation. The effectiveness and safety of the study remains to be verified.

AUTRES USES OF ESSENTIAL OILS

Alongside using essential oils to aid in aromatherapy practices, they is also a viable option for the purposes mentioned above.

They are used as scents and air fresheners for the home, bathroom and clothing. They are commonly used as scents in cosmetic products as well as other natural and homemade products.

They can also be utilized as an alternative to synthetic repellents against mosquitoes, as they are proven to be safe to use in the natural environment. Certain studies conducted using essential oils such as citronella revealed that mosquitoes can be repellent when using these oils. Citronella when combined with vanillin results in an even more effective outcome.

Essential oils can also be utilized to preserve food items. They can also be used to be used in industrial processes.

Chapter 7: Commonly asked questions

This chapter will cover a lot of the concerns you might be asking about essential oils, particularly if you've never previously used them. There are many choices and information to choose from that you could have difficult time deciding on how to use their benefits and how they function. This chapter will cover the various issues and by the end of it, you will be armed with all the information you require to begin.

What are the essential oils that are used?

There are three ways of making use of essential oils. They can be applied directly on the skin, inhaled to release their aroma and in some instances, consumed. While we'll discuss the possibility of inhaling essential oils in some instances, it should only be done under supervision by a certified healthcare provider. If not done correctly, ingesting essential oils can be hazardous.

For inhaling the essential oils there are many methods to achieve this. You can start by using the diffuser. Essential oils are placed inside a diffuser (with the option of water or not, refer to the directions) and it will warm the scent before releasing it in the air. There is no recommendation you directly burn essential oils and this indirect heat method is much better.

The other method you can breathe in essential oil is via dry evaporate. It is as simple as soaking the cotton ball with oil, and leaving it in your vicinity, then the fragrance will spread throughout the air. If you want a stronger scent it is possible to sniff your cotton ball.

Third, some individuals employ steam as a method to disperse the oil. To achieve this, pour 2 or 3 drops in the steaming bowl. Then, drape the towel over the bowl , and inhale the steam. Make sure not to consume excessive amounts of the oil, as it can be a powerful way to make use of the oils, and too much could become excessive.

Another method used to disperse the scent is to add several drops of oil in a solution containing water which is mixed before being spraying in the atmosphere. If you create an oil in this manner and store it in a container ensure that you shake the bottle prior to every use.

Certain essential oils may be consumed. While the majority of internal use of these oils should be done under the supervision of a licensed health practitioner, there is some information in this book regarding the use of essential oils. If you decide to go with this practice of using oils, be sure you receive 100% pure, or food grade essential oils. If you're consuming oils, then you don't have any impurities within your oil. It may cost a little more, but it is no harm for your health. We recommend that you talk about internal usage with a specialist who will be able to guide you in the right direction.

The third approach we will discuss the use of the oils is applying them on the skin. It's important to apply them cautiously, since the oils are extremely potent and some may cause an allergic reaction, particularly for those with sensitive skin. It is crucial to remember that the majority of oils must be dilute before being employed in this manner. The standard rule of thumb is that the ratio of the oil in relation in relation to the substance should be less than three to five percent. A carrier substance is the one that you combine the oil. It is usually water, but could also be a vegetable oil or nuts oil. To give you an idea of how much when you apply just one tablespoon of the water carrier (such in the form of water) then add one drop of a 3- percent solution. The solution is then rub into the skin.

Other methods to utilize essential oils is to use them in a bath or an oil for massage. To use it in a bath take some drops of essential oils in the water just prior to entering. If you suffer from sensitive skin blend oils with carrier oil prior making this preparation (see further below). There are also people who make an Epson salt blend using essential oils. Mix one teaspoon baking soda, 2 Epsom salts and three pieces sea salt. Add six drops of the selected essential oil in the mix before adding it to the bath.

Additionally, it can be used to massage oil. For this, you must be sure that you do not apply more than a one per cent solution. This is 1 drop of oil for each 3 teaspoons (or the equivalent of one teaspoon) of the oil. The oil can be employed for massages.

How can I make use of to use an essential oil diffuser?

In this book, we'll be discussing the process of diffusing the aroma of essential oils in diffusers. There are many kinds of diffusers, however they all accomplish the same function, which is to allow the vapors of the essential oils that you use to penetrate all the surrounding air, so that you reap all the advantages of their scent. Let's review the various kinds of diffusers and the ways they function.

The first is the candle diffuser. If a candle is lit the reservoir is placed above the flame to store your essential oils and the water mix that you're heating. These are easy to use and offer an energizing scent from the oils you use, however they don't usually provide a sufficient amount of the fragrance to offer any significant therapeutic benefit. They should not be used when the use of essential oils for purposes of therapeutic use.

The second kind of diffuser is an electric heat diffuser. They operate by placing oil on a small absorbent pad in an heating chamber. The chamber is then ventilated, which allows the compound to evaporate into the air. This is a fantastic instrument for dispersing heavier oils. It requires minimal maintenance to operate this kind of diffuser. However, excessive heat as that found in this type of diffuser may harm essential oils that are more volatile by altering their chemical composition and rendering them untherapeutic.

The most popular diffuser is the one that most people utilize most often, which is the diffuser that uses cool air to nebulize. This type of diffuser uses the pressure created by a compressor to evaporate the oil essential to air. A glass nebulizing lamp serves as a condenser. It produces a strong therapeutic vapor that is released into the air, without relying on heat, which means that the compounds are not destroyed in order to disperse it. It is the only diffuser that needs regular cleaning and can get tiring. Certain viscous oils, like sandalwood oil and ylang-ylang oil, are not able to diffuse inside these diffusers. You might require an electronic heat diffuser to diffuse these.

There's another type of diffuser you could take with your wherever you go. It is known as diffuser jewelry. There are necklaces, bracelets and other accessories specifically designed for the purpose of storing essential oils for use while on the move. They're similar to lockets that open for you to see a disk you can add a few drops of your favorite oil on , so that the aroma is accessible throughout the time of the day. It's much simpler to carry essential oils on your person.

Where can I purchase essential oil items?

There are numerous reputable suppliers of essential oils and are located in a variety of municipalities and in towns. Natural sites, healing clinics and aromatherapy shops are available in a variety of locations. Make sure that the company you purchase at is well-informed and offering high-quality products, particularly those oils as well as other components in the preparation of recipes. It is more crucial when the oil you're using is consumed by any means.

What safety precautions should I follow prior to making use of essential oils?

Essential oils are highly potent, therefore there are some things to know prior to making use of essential oils.

Before you start, perform first a test on the skin of the oil. Some people are sensitive to skin and may not be able to cope well with direct contact with skin. If you are one of them you should opt for an inhalation method to use the oil. It is obvious that if you are sensitized to oils applied to your skin, don't apply it. Also, don't let the oil get in your eyes. Thirdly, ensure that you purchase the best quality oils. You don't want to buy oils that have other contaminants in them. When you apply an oil and do not feel well following the use it is best to stop using it. You need to determine if something makes you feel great or not. If you don't then it's time to stop using it. Be sure to trust your gut.

Remember that the majority of essential oils need to be dilute. Avoid using them directly unless the directions on the bottle suggest it. If in doubt try diluting it.

What percentage of essential oil should I apply?

There is less to be had in the case of essential oils. Start with a single drop and observe how it affects you. You may increase the amount the amount however, if you begin with excessive amounts, you could be a victim of some negative effects. Some recipes or instructions could require a different approach and you must follow these guidelines.

What should I look out for when buying essential oils?

Make sure you purchase the highest quality oils you can locate. If you can, look for oils that aren't altered or altered in any manner. Pure oils are the best provided you understand how to use them correctly (which we've already talked about). The reason is that you want to avoid unfamiliar additives to your oils that might not be beneficial.

Then, ensure that you are getting oils from plants that were grown organically. If the plant was grown using pesticides, they can be transferred to oils. Make sure the oils have been examined for purity before they are offered for sale. If you can't locate the data on the label, it is posted on the company's website. Being aware that this product was tested to detect contamination can be very calming on the mind.

Finding the highest essential oils of the highest quality is among the best ways to improve your well-being.

What is the definition of a carrier oil?

Essential oils are extremely potent when applied directly. Carrier oils are an oil that is blended with essential oils in order to reduce the potent substances. Most often, water is utilized in this case, however in the event that the oil is blended in with another, the other oil is referred to as a carrier.

There are many different oils that are utilized to make carrier oils. Here are some of the most popular carrier oils, and the characteristics they offer:

Grapeseed oil is lightweight and thin, making it ideal for massage oils as well as moisturizing. It's a little bit short in shelf time.

Sweet Almond Oil has a sweet and nutty scent and can be used for use as a carrier oil that can be used in a variety of ways. Avoid using this oil in the case of an allergy to nuts.

Jojoba oil has a slight sweet nutty scent and an appearance that is similar to the natural oils of your skin, making it non-greasy skin. Also, it has a long shelf life.

Olive oil is simple to purchase at your local supermarket, however it comes with a thick oily consistency, powerful smell, and a brief shelf time. It's popular because it is available in every grocery store.

The fractionated coconut oil can be boiled into a solid at the room temperatures (unlike normal coconut oil) and is odorless and is therefore better when mixed with essential oils as it doesn't alter the scent. It doesn't feel oily to the touch and also has an extremely long shelf time.

Coconut oil that is regular in its composition liquid at ambient temperature, and has a coconut scent (unlike it is a fractionated oil). It also has a long shelf-life and gives a moisturizing, oily feel on the skin after applying.

The shea butter can be a solid when it's at the room temperature, and it has a distinct nutty scent. It is commonly used to moisturize skin and gives a waxy feel to the skin.

Cocoa butter is substance that is solid when it's at room temperature. However, many find it hard to handle, which is why it's not the best choice as carrier oil. Most of the time, it is mixed along with various oils.

Certain recipes might require various carrier oils. These are the most frequently employed carriers and must keep in your pantry.

Do I need to be using essential oils while pregnant or for children?

If you're pregnant there are some essential oils to be avoiding. This includes basil, cassia the cinnamon bark Sage lemongrass, rosemary thyme, vetiver and white forested.

Additionally, there are some things you shouldn't do be doing when using essential oils during pregnancy. Be extremely cautious in your first trimester. A significant amount of the development of the fetus takes place during this period, which is why it is essential to be particularly cautious the way you apply essential oils. Additionally, you must dilute essential oils prior to you use them during pregnancy. Thirdly, if not sure, use them to aid in aromatherapy to inhale the scent like we have mentioned previously. Most of the worry about essential oils stems from the external and topical use of the oils. If you have any concerns seek out an expert on essential oils.

Essential oils safe to use during breastfeeding include clary, bergamot the sage, grapefruit, geranium lavender, lemon patchesouli, melaleuca sandalwood, roman chamomile wild orange and ylang-ylang. It is important to remember that peppermint may decrease the quantity of milk in your breast therefore, use it in small amounts while nursing.

For youngsters, you can apply essential oils to treat their skin, but it's crucial to remember that you should apply them in much more diluted forms than for an adult who is healthy. They should be dilute by twice the amount you do as an adult and use them at a quarter strength for use for babies. Essential oils can cause harm for children, particularly when they are taken in large quantities. Another thing to remember is that what you must apply essential oils for children is to apply them on the bottoms of feet. Since the skin is more thick there, it causes less irritation.

What's the main difference between aromatherapy oils and essential oils?

This is a crucial concern. There's a significant difference between them, and you must be aware. In general, an aromatherapy oil is two percent strength of an essential oil , with more than 98 percent made up of either grapeseed or almond oil. The carrier and the oil generally are not of high quality and could be extremely expensive for the amount you're buying.

In contrast essential oils are pure and does not mix with other substances. Additionally, if you're purchasing a top-quality product you won't have to worry about the presence of contamination within the oil.

When purchasing essential oils, make sure it's labeled "Pure essential oil." If it's not labeled with a different name then it's not truly pure. You may also visit the website of the company for information on the purity test and the quality of the oil.

What should I do to store My Essential Oils?

There are a few points to keep in mind when you are keeping essential oils in your home to ensure that they continue to remain efficient. It is important to keep them well-nourished and have the best potency, therefore, to achieve this follow these steps. Make sure the oils are stored in dark colored bottles because the glass used for storage will remove ultraviolet rays from the light source that could cause the oils to degrade. Be sure to never let your oils exposed to direct sunlight. Place them in a dry, cool area. Oils exposed to frequent, drastic variations in temperature will reduce the quality of the oil faster. To keep the oils in good condition longer, it's recommended to store them in a dark, cool place. If you've got room to store them, put them in the refrigerator. Certain oils with carriers could be able to solidify in these cold temperatures, but you are able to gradually warm the oil prior to using it.

It is also important to keep carriers oils inside the refrigerator especially during season of summer, to avoid loss of the oils. If you are unable to store them in the refrigerator There are boxes that you can keep your carrier oils and oils in, to ensure they stay cool and dry.

It is equally important to keep the carriers and oils away from spark sources and open flames since these are extremely volatile and could spark. They can be highly flammable.

Be sure to secure the cap on your containers in the event that you do not use them, to ensure they do not evaporate.

Don't keep oils that are not dilute within plastic bottle. The oils may be absorbed by the bottles and make the bottles melt. Low concentrations of diluted oils could be kept in bottles made of plastic.

How do essential oils last? How long can they be kept?

The shelf duration of essential oils can differ greatly based on the oil, its storage space it is stored in and many other aspects. The most crucial thing is possible to do in order to maintain the potency of essential oils is to store them in a dark, cool space, in the manner described earlier.

If you follow the guidelines regarding storage, the majority of essential oils will be able to last two years. However, the exception is the fact that tea tree and fir oils last between 12 and 18 months. The same goes for cold-pressed citrus oils are expected to last for 9-12 months.

Essential oils aren't rancid or discolor. Instead, they diminish the therapeutic properties they possess as well as chemical chain reaction reactions alter the ingredients that are effective in the oils.

The typical carrier oil shelf life of 9 to 15 months. Grapeseed oil is the one with the longest shelf life of all, lasting 6 - 9 months. Unlike essential oils, carrier oils do turn rancid. Carrier oils are more susceptible to temperature changes, and it is essential to store them properly.

The best option is to purchase the essential oils in smaller quantities so that they can be replaced and replenished regularly. This can solve the issue of whether the oils are useful.

Now that you've got the fundamental information is required to begin using oil-based essentials, it's time to get into the oils that are needed to help you lose weight. In the next section, you will contain all the details you require to start losing weight using essential oils!

Chapter 8: Choosing the Essential Oil That's Right for You

The ideal essential oil to purchase depends on three factors such as the purpose, budget and your personal preferences.

The purpose

It was stated within the intro that essential oils could be utilized for a variety of issues. The majority of people purchase bottles of essential oils just for one reason however it is important to be aware of the many benefits the essential oil has.

To make it easier for you, this chapter will explain the reason for the study and then provide the essential oils that can be utilized for that.

Anti-bacterial to treat wounds, skin infections and acne in humans and pet animals (topically applied) The ingredients are lavender and peppermint, eucalyptus, tea tree oil

Antibacterial essential oils can also be used to disinfect your home.

Relaxing/Reduces stress/Helps with insomnia (inhaled scent) Lavender, chamomile Geranium, vetiver sandalwood, tangerine and vanilla

Cleans noses that are stuffed (inhaled scent) The scents include Peppermint, lavender, eucalyptus,

Removes dark spots from the face (topically applied) Lemon, chamomile and rose

Clears dandruff: tea tree oil, eucalyptus, peppermint

It reduces itching particularly for eczema and psoriasis (topically applied) such as peppermint, lavender, eucalyptus oil

Kills fleas, ticks, and lice in pet and humans (topically applied) The ingredients are lavender peppermint, eucalyptus tea tree oil

Concentration increases (inhaled scent) Inhale jasmine, peppermint

Enhances your energy levels (inhaled scent) Grapefruit, lemon and lime

Enhances metabolism (when taken in) Includes: ginger, cinnamon grapefruit, lemon, peppermint

stimulates blood flow to epidermis for the regeneration of skin as well as hair growth (topically applied) Lavender and peppermint. Rose Geranium, sandalwood vanilla, rosemary

It is important to note that many essential oils serve many different purposes. This is why it's feasible to cut costs making use of essential oils. There is no requirement to purchase separate products for different requirements. Furthermore, since essential oils are in essence, concentrated (unless they're labeled as dilute) and only a tiny amount is needed each time. A bottle of 30 milliliters that costs $10 could last for one year, depending on how it is utilized.

Also, note that lavender may be used to serve a variety of functions. That's why it's known as the most universal essential oil. It is also considered to be the most safe to use. The allergy to lavender is extremely rare and most people suffering from medical conditions can benefit from it. (However it is important to note that, as previously mentioned people with medical issues should talk to their doctor first in order to be sure they are on the safe side , even if they just use lavender.)

Budget

As previously mentioned essential oils can differ in cost due to a variety of reasons. It is the responsibility of the user to decide if the extra cost is worth the cost. Be aware that the more expensive essential oil isn't typically more efficient. In this case both rose and lavender essential oils work well for facial rejuvenation, however the rose essential oil is costlier since there are more plants needed for the production of the equivalent amount of essential oil. But, as each person's body is unique it is possible that one's personal experience could be able to prove that rose is superior to lavender in this particular case, so the higher cost is worth it.

Personal Preferences

Of of course, people always decide what they prefer to use. If you have found that both rose and lavender are effective , but you prefer the fragrance of roses and lavender, it is sensible to purchase rose essential oils instead.

Chapter 9: Depression and Anxiety Essential Oil Recipes

The recipes included in this chapter can be helpful in times of stress, depressed , or just want energy or energy. If you are using essential oils, especially first time, be sure to follow the safety guidelines on the bottle. Check to see if the oils are safe for use on the skin prior to applying them to your skin.

Mood Enhancing Blends of Oils to Create:

Blues Banishing Blend No. One:

To make this blend, mix with the orange essential oil with three drops essential oil for sandalwood as well as 1 drop rose essential oil.

Anxiety-Reducing Blend No. 2:

This recipe calls for two drops of clary Sage oil and three drops the oil of bergamot.

A Mood Lifting Mixture Number Three

To make this mix to make it, mix three drops grapefruit oil One drop of lavender along with one drop flower oil.

Happiness Inducing Recipe #4:

To make a mood-lifting blend Mix two drops of Jasmine Oil, 2 drops lemon oil as well as two drops of the oil of frankincense.

Mood Enhancing Blend Five

Combine five drops lavender oil and 2 drops patchouli along with four drops lemongrass oil to create a stress-busting recipe.

The recipes can be utilized in many ways. Once you've crafted each of these recipes select a specific mix and apply it to one possible manner:

Strategies to Make Use of these Mixtures:

Make use of an oil diffuser:

It is possible to create your own diffuser-ready blend by following the recipe above simply by multiplying each ingredient with four. Then, you add the ingredients into the glass bottle and mix it with a shaker or rolling it around in your hands. After that, you'll include the recommended amount of drops of oil you have chosen from the blend you have created to the oil diffuser you decide to make use of. Follow the directions on the instruction manual for your oil diffuser.

Make use of the Blend in the Bath:

Whatever your particular need An aromatic bath is an excellent method to satisfy your requirements. Combine one of the recipes mentioned above to get the mood-boosting benefits you're looking for. You can also mix oils to get additional benefits.

Mix your Oil Recipe using Bath Salts Mix Your Oil Recipe with Bath Salts buy bath salts at the supermarket and mix the oil blend you prefer to them to enhance the fragrance and moisturizing properties for your skin.

Include the Oils in the Carrier Oil to create a relaxing massage Blend:

Olive oil, almond oil or jojoba are all suitable to relax your muscles. Mix the blend you prefer to any of these oils to create an energizing and relaxing massage. To get the most relaxing benefits warm it in the microwave approximately 10 seconds.

A dark mood doesn't have to be a source of stress. Begin using fantastic essential oils, made from natural ingredients to fight the blues. Begin to connect with nature and begin improving your life today by making your own oils.

Chapter 10: Holistic Uses

A disclaimer of sorts before we begin: don't under any circumstance substituting essential oils or other holistic therapies for prescribed medications without consulting your physician first.

If you're pregnant, consult your physician to confirm that the essential oil that you are considering trying is suitable for you and your baby.

If you're taking any medication it is advisable to speak with your physician to find out if specific essential oils react to that medication in a negative way.

You're likely to be fine, but it's prudent to check with your doctor before taking any new supplements, whether holistic or not. Being cautious is a good idea all the time in regards to your health.

However holistic methods are a great, natural alternative to treat mild conditions and providing preventative treatment. Since they are tiny in molecular size , and are Lipid-soluble (which means they are taken up by the skin) They have the capability to heal at the level of the cellular by entering cells' walls. In just 20 minutes they could be affecting every cell of your body.

Essential oils can also be readily metabolized by other nutrients, meaning that they do not accumulate within the body. They simply do what they are supposed to and then leave like they're not there.

Therapy with Oxygen

Essential oils contain oxygen. They aid in transporting nutrition throughout the body. It aids in stimulating the immune system, as diseases begin when cells are deficient in oxygen in order to properly assimilate nutrients.

Snoring, Sinuses, Antioxidants and Snoring:

Essential oils also contain powerful antioxidants that boost your immune system, preventing the attack of free radicals. They also fight fungi, which assists with a range of ailments.

Colds: Lavender Eucalyptus, Rosemary (these are best if they are combined with the cream or milk. Put them in an icy bath)

Fevers: Eucalyptus, Peppermint, Lavender (also recommended to use in baths)

Sinus problems: Fir Needle (apply a 50/50 dilution of your chest)

Snoring Affair: Thyme (apply 50/50 dilution on the soles of your feet prior to you go to bed)

Combating Infections: Cuts or bruises, bumps, bruises and Parasites:

Certain essential oils are antibacterial as well as anti-fungal, antitumoral, Anti-parastic and antimicrobial. This means they are able to kill bacteria and viruses combating illnesses and helping to restore health. They also have anti-carcinogenic properties this means they can be extremely effective in fighting certain cancers and in preventing them.

Some of the most essential oils to accomplish this include:

Bruises: Clove, Lavender

Ringworm It is a unique recipe that requires 3 drops of Tea Tree, 3 drops of Spearmint oil, 1 drop of Peppermint and one drop Rosemary. Mix these ingredients with 10 drops of carrier oil and apply the mixture on the designated zone between two and four times a every day.

Cuts and scrapes: Clove, Lavender, Tea Tree

Stings and Insect Bite: Lavender, Peppermint, Wintergreen

Detoxifying

Since they pass through capillaries, and eventually into the bloodstream essential oils are effective in detoxifying your body that cleanse cells and bloodstream and helping to restore balance to your overall well-being.

Weight Loss

Certain essential oils, such as Coriander can aid in breaking down fats via hydrolysis. Other oils, such as Elemi, Hyssop, Lemon, Myrrh, and Myrtle can help tighten and tone your muscles.

A few studies have also proven that by inhaling the oil of peppermint (using the secure methods explained in the book) it can help you reduce calories more quickly.

Mental Health and Brain Health

Certain essential oils have sesquiterpenes (compounds which deliver oxygen-rich molecules into cells). Sesquiterpenes remove and/or reprogram faulty code in the cellular memory. This is why medical experts believe they can be beneficial in the fight against cancer and other diseases. In doing so they also make it difficult the cancerous cells from reproducing. They sucker punch them on the face, to put it that way.

This is particularly beneficial for the health of your brain.

There is a part of your brain that is known as a blood-brain barrier. The barrier acts as a filter that only those molecules with a weight of lesser than 800-1000 amu (amu) to travel to the brain.

This is both beneficial as well as bad. It's a good thing as it prevents harmful substances from entering your brain. It's not good because, should you are diagnosed with cancer of the brain, chemotherapy will not be effective because the blood-brain barrier blocks out the majority of drugs, rendering the treatment unusable.

Essential oils consist from molecules with a weight of less than 500 amu. This means they can are able to pass through the blood brain barrier, and carry the remarkable anti-cancer properties of their sesquiterpenes along with them.

They also have lipid-soluble and can get through the barrier without difficulty.

Because of this essential oils are beneficial in the treatment of Alzheimer's, Cancer, Lou Gehrig's Disease, Multiple Sclerosis and Parkinson's Disease.

They also assist with headaches, memory issues migraines, anxiety tension, and a variety of other conditions affecting mental and emotional balance.

These are some of the best appropriate ways to use essential oils with regard to mental and physical health:

For headaches:Peppermint, Wintergreen, Roman Chamomile or Spearmint (apply 2 drops, diluted, on the back of your neck, behind your ears, on your temples, on your forehead and under your nose). It is also possible to apply Lavender to treat tension headaches.

For focus and memory: Calamus, Ginger, or Rosemary

To treat anxiousness: Basil, Calamus, Camphor, Chamomile, Clary Sage, Clove, Davana, Dill, Lavender, Manuka, Melissa, Mugwort, Myrtle, Neroli, Patchouli as well as Valerian (This one is the best for preventing teeth grinding. Apply 3 drops on the soles of your feet prior to when you go to sleep in the evening).

As a treatment for depression: Bergamot Birch, Cassia, Chamomile, Citronella, Davana, Grapefruit, Jasmine, Lavandin, Lemongrass, Melissa, Neroli Patchouli, Peppermint or Ylang-Ylang.

For insomnia: Calamus Cypress, Dill, Frankincense, Jasmine, Lavender, Lemongrass, Mandarin, Marjoram, Mullein, or Roman Chamomile

For Fatigue: Birch, Boldo, Cassia, Camphor, Elemi, or Peppermint,

For sexual health: Jasmine, Mugwort, or Patchouli

Skin Health:

This differs from normal skin treatment (which is covered in the cosmetic section of the book). Essential oils can ease sunburns, rashes, and other skin-related conditions.

The most important essential oils to have around for such occasions are:

Sunburns Lavender, Rose, and Roman Chamomile (Disclaimer These are all beneficial only if it's one-degree burns without any obvious blisters. If your sunburn is much more than that, visit the doctor and inquire the treatments available.) The most effective method to treat sunburns using essential oils would be to use two drops (diluted by carrier oil) and then soak an unwashed cotton ball. Utilize the sponge to spread the oil on the area that is inflamed.

Poison Oak/Poison Ivy The most common is peppermint or Wintergreen (apply three drops dispersed with a carrier oil two times a day)

Nausea, Aches and Pains:

Drinking hangovers Juniper Berry Cedarwood, Grapefruit, Lavender, Rosemary or Lemon (Use 6-8 drops of each one of them in bath)

Improved Circulation: Mix eight to ten drops Neroli in your bath. It is also beneficial to mix the Neroli with some Epson salt first.

The causes of nausea are: Peppermint, Patchouli, Ginger or Nutmeg

Menstrual Cramps Clary Sage, Basil, Rosemary or Sage

Muscle and Joint Pain Birch, Basil, Copaida, Cypress, Elemi, Eucalyptus, Lemongrass, Patchouli, Peppermint, Sage, Vetiver or Wintergreen

The most common strains are Basil, Kanuka, Pine or Wintergreen (apply 3-4 times a day)

Chapter 11: The Precautions to Be aware of prior to using essential oils

Essential oils are extremely concentrated volatile oils. As an instance, it is required to consume up to 150 pounds lavender flowers to create one 1 pound in lavender essential oil.Similarly 1 drop of peppermint essential oil is comparable to drinking 25-28 cup in peppermint tea.That means that a small of peppermint oil can go a very far distance which is one reason why essential oils are offered in small bottles.The higher concentration produces a higher levels of medicinal properties too.Just as painkillers, which have specific precautions regarding the amount that is safe to use for 24 hours and essential oils shouldn't be used excessively either.This isn't to say that essential oils shouldn't be utilized, however, essential oils should only be used after you have been educated about their usage and the benefits.

In addition to inhaling essential oils, applying essential oils that are not diluted on your skin could pose dangers as well.Because the essential oils' molecules are tiny, these molecules can easily get into your skin and in your bloodstream.However the use of the use of a carrier liquid or lotion and diluting essential oil is generally a way to lower the possibility of irritation on the skin or an allergic reaction.Essential oils should not be applied to the skin, undiluted, with only certain exceptions, and only under the supervision of an authorized aromatherapist.For each 3-5 drops of oil, you must use 1 tsp to 1TBSP of solid or liquid carrier, such as coconut oil or almond.

If you are using citrus oils on the skin, remember that they can cause your skin to become more sensitive towards the sun.There are some components in the oils that cause UV rays more vulnerable to penetrate your skin's protective layer which can lead to skin discoloration, blisters and burning.The most commonly used "photosensitive" (most susceptible to making your skin sensitive to sun) oils are citrus lemon, lime grapefruit and bergamot.

For individuals that are elderly, pregnant, children or babies, extreme caution should be used when applying essential oils.Several different essential oils can cause blood pressure to increase, or certain beneficial bacteria in your gut to be killed.It is best to check with a qualified aromatherapist.Lavender is generally safe for most individuals, including children and babies, however make sure this essential oil is very diluted before applying.

Essential oils are hazardous.Not solely are essential oils flammable, and shouldn't be used to treat eye problems However, certain plant materials shouldn't be used or used in the form of vital oils.The National Association of Aromatherapy will assist you in finding an aromatherapist and describing the essential oils to never ever be used.However the essential oils can be safe if used with respect and correctly.They are potent therapeutic ingredients, and can offer relief from numerous illnesses, yet they can trigger many problems if misused.

Chapter 12: What's That? A Guide To Essential Oils

The essential oils are in use since the beginning of the age of. Since the day an individual realized that plants can be utilized to do more than just eat and could be beneficial in saving the life of someone else essential oils have been in use.

In the past, pharmacies were the modern equivalent to hospitals. They were the place to go for tooth that was in pain or you could not overcome a cough has been bothering you for a while. When you visit the Apothecary, you could receive an treatment for almost everything that was bothering you.

Sometimes, it works, but sometimes it did not.

Remember, in the past the people still spread maggots and poop on their open wounds. However, there was some things they discovered through trial and trial and. The most reliable historical evidence of the essential oils used throughout Western time is from The Islamic Nations that rose up in the Middle Ages.

Also, keep in mind that Islamic kingdoms and countries that arose in the Middle Ages made most of Europe appear like primitive people. They weren't smashing rocks. They documented the healing properties of specific plants, flowers, roots and leaves which could help treat various ailments or ease the symptoms plaguing those affected by them.

But if you truly would like to meet people who were aware of the art of doing things then you should look at China or to the Far East. Eastern Medicine has endured to today and is possibly the most ancient form of use in pharmaceuticals for natural cures and methods of healing. It is possible to look at countries like China, India, and Japan which have a long study of and practice of using plants and other natural ingredients to treat diseases that impact the body.

As technology has advanced and newer and better solutions are developed for old issues essential oils have remained in use. In the event of natural catastrophes, or when shortages happen during times of warfare, plague or famine, natural remedies located in the forest, gardens and deserts around the world are can be found to aid us. Instead of taking an e-cigarette that will harm your liver over the course of time, why not try some natural and organic remedies to ease your pain.

If you're looking for a more detailed explanation of what they are?

The essential oils are extracted from the bark, leaves roots, any other plant part which has been proven to possess medicinal properties. Certain plants possess multiple essential oils, but the majority don't. For instance, you'll take the leaf of oregano in order to extract the essential oils from it but not the root system , nor the stem. In contrast you'll pick the orange's peel and the fruit of an orange and the blossom of an orange tree in order to get essential oils from them all.

The majority of essential oils are broken down into different properties or parts of the plant or tree that are used the most. They are classified as flowers, berries and bark leaves, peels, resin, rhizome seeds, wood, and. There is a good chance to see each essential oil split down into these different sources within the plant. The methods used to extract essential oils from these plant parts is a bit more difficult.

In the past the only way to extract the oils from an object of plant material was by the act of expression or, as we refer to it as crushing. They would have two large flat surfaces and would smash them together, effectively pressing the oils out along alongside the other liquids. They would then collect it by putting it into water. Oil is deposited on top of the water, and they then remove it by skimming it off.

We've evolved to be to a greater extent than simply squeeze things. Nowadays, distillation is the most commonly used method of extracting essential oils. Those who do not use distillation employ solvents to extract those essential oils. It's a complicated and lengthy process, but in final, it functions as a charm.

What is taken is really nothing more than pure essence from the plants. It's the smell of the plant at its most pure form. And it is extremely harmful and deadly when you come into contact with it without diluting or making sure you take care of it appropriately.

In fact, you may be causing serious harm when you apply it to your skin , or coming into contact with your mouth or eyes. However, experts take care of the essentials and ensure that the product you'll purchase is safe and effective for you.

Now knowing what the is essential oil, what do they benefit you and how will they help improve your well-being? Let me provide the details.

Chapter 13: Lavender Essential Oil

Name: Lavender

Scientific Name: Lavandula anguvstifolia and Lavandula officinalis

Cost: The average price is $15 for one ounce of organic lavender oil

Essential oils have experienced an increase in their demand because knowledge about the benefits of aromatherapy and holistic medical treatments have become more accessible to the general public. Lavender is one of the most popular, well-known and easily accessible of the vast range of beneficial essential oils. The oil is extracted through distillation of flower spikes of certain species, this aromatic and healing oil offers a myriad of advantages.

Essential oil of lavender has been documented as helping humans for over two thousand years as evidenced by Egyptians, Phoenicians and several other civilizations using the oil to aid in processes ranging that range from Mummification, a sacred ritual to a treatment for insomnia. Even Romans consider lavender to be an expensive commodity, frequently selling for more than 100 denarii (the most commonly used measure of the roman currency) per pounds. The scent was used for bathing houses, insect repellent and even to flavor food it, it cost the equivalent of one month's wage for an agricultural worker.

In the Renaissance the time of the Renaissance, lavender was spread across the damp, cold floors of castles to serve as disinfectant and deodorant in addition to enjoying widespread use in the gardens of apothecaries. The lavender flower experienced a second rise in popularity in the period of plague, and it was customary to attach small bouquets of lavender to the wrists to protect against the highly anticipated Black Death. In addition, its capability to repel pests was instrumental in helping fight off diseases and pestilence.

In the past few years the flower has been shown to have been scientifically confirmed to have positive effects. Its role to repel bugs remains just as effective in the present century, just like it was centuries ago there are numerous studies that show it repels mosquitoesand midges, and the majority of moth species. In the event of an insect biting that is not scared by the smell of the oil, lavender has anti-inflammatory properties that alleviate the pain and irritation that usually go together with bites from insects.

The plant's applications go well beyond its capability to deter bugs. Lavender is still frequently used as a remedy for insomnia. Numerous studies on patients with a history of dementia have revealed an increase in the regulation of their sleep cycles once the essential oil was replaced by the prescribed sleep medication. It is generally believed by research circles that it is due to the effect of the flower upon the nerve system. Lavender regulates heart rate as well as improving cognitive performance and bringing about the ideal combination of clarity of thinking and easing stress. This sympathetic response has proved beneficial in the treatment of headaches, migraines, discomfort, and emotional and nervous stress. It does this without the harmful chemicals found in many popular over-the-counter remedies.

The neurological effect permits the oil to be used as a potent treatment for various body discomforts and pains, such as muscles that are tight or sore or joints, rheumatisms, sprains and strains. Massages using lavender essential oil can help relieve joint pain. A study conducted in postoperative pain relief discovered that mixing lavender oil vapor into breathing masks of patients dramatically decreased the level of pain when compared to those who were revived by oxygen purified after the operation.

The breath mask study led to additional discoveries regarding lavender's capacity to treat different respiratory issues, such as throat illnesses, flu, colds as well as sinus congestion, asthma as well as bronchitis, whooping cold and laryngitis to tonsillitis. The oil is used as an oil that is applied to the neck's skin or chest or added to inhalers or vaporizers that are used to treat coughs and colds. The stimulating qualities the essential oils of lavender may help to break up the phlegm sucked within the respiratory tract and reduce congestion caused by breathing issues. The increased oxygen supply and the elimination of phlegm containing germs, could accelerate the process of recovery and aid the body to naturally rid itself of other toxins. The essential lavender oil is also believed to have an antibacterial effect that helps fight respiratory tract infections.

As it continues to benefit its hormones, Lavender essential oil is exceptionally effective in treating urinary issues, as it increases the production of urine and also restores hormonal balance. It has also been proven to ease inflammation and cystitis of the bladder, in both genders, as well being able to ease cramps in females.

However, the Lavender essential oil's benefits aren't only internal. Aromatherapists and dermatologists have rated lavender among the best oils to treat acne through regulating sebum's over-excretion through hormone manipulation. By adding a tiny amount of essential lavender oil into your routine will help to reduce acne as well as help heal and stop the formation of scars over time.

Lavender's usage within the cosmetic industry isn't restricted to the removal of the appearance of blemishes. It is also utilized for natural hair care since it has been demonstrated to neutralize lice and lice eggs and the nits. Additionally, lavender oil may be extremely beneficial in treating hair loss, specifically for those who suffer with Alopecia, (an autoimmune disease which causes the body to reject hair follicles that belong to it). According to an Sottish study "more than 40 percent of Alopecia patients noticed an increase in the growth of their hair when they applied lavender essential oil onto their scalps."

The list of benefits for physical health isn't complete by assisting digestion, fighting cancer and leucorrhoea. Only one thing could outweigh the benefits that lavender oil has is the method to use the treatment. The most straightforward and accessible method to use this oil would be to rub two or three drops in your palms, and then take a slow, deep inhale. The aroma is pulled up to the amygdala nerve for the fastest calming effect to the whole body.

Another option is to apply a tiny amount on the areas of the wrists, temples, and feet.

The most important thing to consider is the diffusion device that disperses essential oils into the air that can be breathed in naturally , breaking down the liquid into tiny molecules. The various types include ultrasonic, cold air heat diffusers, and evaporator. Prices for these little machines differ by region and also by brand. The best method to secure one is to visit the local store for holistic products or go online to purchase.

The most popular application is through aromatherapy in massage. This oil can be mixed into the massage therapist's lotion , and utilized during the session and then applied over the entire face.

Spiritual Values of Lavender

Cleopatra is believed to use the scent of lavender when she was making love potions.It is believed that she lured Julius

Caesar with it and Mark Antony some time after. People living in the regions that border Italy as well as Spain were reported to have used lavender to prevent "evil eyes" (also known as malochia). Tuscans were known to give their children lavender for protection. It is also believed to protect against illness particularly serious ones like the Black Death. Many of the stories that have been told about lavender are based on protection and love.

I, along with other spiritual healers I have met and across time have utilized lavender the most frequently for the followingreasons:

Heart issues

Protection under various conditions

In order to improve communication, particularly in interviews and relationships.

Help with sleep problems like insomnia and nightmares

Relax and rejuvenate the body, mind, and soul

To stimulate the ability to think clearly

To ease the harsh spiritual energies of animals or people

The spiritual uses of lavender generally are correlated with the colour of the plant as well as the planet with which it is located and, in this case the the planet Mercury. The lavender plant is believed to resonate more than average humans, and therefore raise the frequency of your life.

The methods of spiritual and medicinal use can be utilized to treat a variety of diseases mentioned, and can provide fast relief. So do not be afraid to experiment with the methods that work best for you. The last ten years have proven the numerous benefits of this beneficial flower and we are able to anticipate what the next ten years will reveal.

On the next page you'll find a variety of helpful recipes to help you deal with different conditions.Please make sure to use them in a responsible manner and modify them according to your personal needs.Remember they are just suggestions. Once you are more comfortable with how you and the environment react to lavender it will become easier to adjust the characteristics of the essential oil to suit your requirements.

Recipe for Lavender Linen Mist

1. Include 20-30 drops Lavender Essential oil for 1.5 tablespoons of distillation water into the spray bottle.

2. Mix thoroughly.

3. Lightly mist the bedding. Don't spray so much that it makes them damp as bedsheets that are damp tend to be uncomfortable.

4. Shake well prior to use.

Recipe for Lavender House Cleansing Spray

1. Purchase an 8oz bottle

2. Include 1 oz Witch Hazel to the bottle

3. Incorporate 20-30 drops Lavender Essential Oil

4. Add water distilled until the bottle is about filled

5. Close the shaker and shake it well.

6. Allow to cure in a dark, cool location for 3-4 weeks or until the mixture is fully mature.

The recipe for Lavender Essential Oil Acne and Scar Remedy

1. Obtain amber glass dropper bottle

2. Add 1 tablespoon of jojoba oil (or your preferred carrier oil)

3. Add 5 drops Lavender Essential Oil

4. Add 2 drops of Lemon Essential Oil.

5. Cover the bottle with a lid and shake the bottle to mix oils.

6. Use 2-3 drops of mixture to the area affected and spread uniformly

7. Shake well prior to each use.

Lavender Purification Bath Ritual

Mix 30-40 drops Lavender essential oil to the water in a tub that is lukewarm.

Take a bath and start to breath deeply.Inhale for seven counts. Exhale for hold for 7 seconds and exhale to count 7.

Make a prayer of cleansing according to your belief system. It could be an affirmation such as "I am clean and free from all physical, mental and spiritual energy that prevents in my pursuit of living the most fulfilling life. I am liberated." You could also pray a prayer like that of the 23rd Psalm. Be aware of what you are saying.

Imagine a glowing lavender light shining through the water and over your entire body. Feel it moving through your body, purifying you of anything that is not yours to you, or anything that doesn't bring you happiness.

Pray a prayer of praise for the work that has been done. Trust that this was accomplished for you.

Utilizing your hands rub the body's surface from bottom to top, using the lavender bath water seven times.

Take yourself out of the tub immediately and wash the tub using the lavender Spray for cleaning your home.

Recipe for Lavender Peace & Protection Oil

Mix 20 drops of the oil with 2 oz Olive Oil

Make sure you apply a coat of oil on the top of each door that you have in your home

A few drops can be added to every corner of your home.

A few drops of the oil can be added onto the steering wheel your vehicle

Sprinkle a few drops on your work desk

A few drops can be added onto your shoe's interior as well as your carry around in your purse or wallet

Make the Lord's Prayer, or make an affirmation like "Everywhere I put this oil , it is instantly full of security, peace and love. This is exactly what it is."

Recipe for Lavender Love Attraction Oil

Incorporate 20 drops of lavender essential oil as well as a few floral lavender to 2oz Sweet almond oil.

Call upon the spirits, angels and ancestors who most evoke the kind of love you wish to boost. Relax your eyes, and sense their presence. It's helpful to smile.

Three drops should be placed between each ear, across all Chakra points.See my Chakra book if you're not acquainted with Chakras. Repeat this every day until you feel the love you desire to improve your life.

Ritual to Lavender Daily Protection

Simply apply Lavender Essential Oil on your wrists, your temples and inner thighs, as well as your lower back, neck back and behind your ear to shield yourself from negative or unwelcome energies, and to attract positive thinking, high-frequency people.

Lavender is among the most adaptable and popular essential oils that exist in both the metaphysical and medical communities. It's an adaptogenic oil, meaning it helps the body deal with stress better and the restoration of the normal physiological stress levels better (Webster's Dictionary.) It's antiviral and an antiseptic, and also antibacterial. Here are 15 more ways to make use of lavender oil.

15 Physical Benefits of Lavender Essential Oil

Create a lavender-scented dream pillow to sleep better. add 20 drops of lavender in 1 cups of lavender dried. Create a pouch made of silk and then add to it the mixture.Close the pouch, then place it under your mattress.

Clean and energize both antique and brand new items , as well as modern items in your home

Apply it behind the ear and mix it with coconut oil to nourish your body.

Apply it to the nose to soothe or prevent colds as well as sinus problems

Apply this to the chest to help relieve chest colds and asthma issues.

Apply the humidifier on your body to help soothe the symptoms of cold and asthma.

Add sweet almonds or jojoba oil , and apply to face for healing acne.

Mix it with tea tree oil Add Brown sugar, jojoba oils and use as scrub for your back to avoid back acne.

Apply the oil to burns, cuts and bites to relieve pain and prevent infection. It also helps promote healing. It is believed that applying lavender to an insect bite can prevent the spread of lyme disease.

Get your mind clear by inhaling the aroma of lavender oil

Apply it to sunburns for soothing and heal.

Mix lavender essential oil with olive oil and brown sugar to make a luxurious body polish

Apply the application to cold sores to help soothe and speed up healing.

Make the bath for feet along the apple cider vinegar for healing foot fungus

Mix it with witch hazel to make an instant body spray to prevent hot flashes

10 Spiritual Uses Additional to Lavender Essential Oil (Metaphysical Aromatherapy)

Utilize lavender to help promote the possibility of prophetic dreams.Simply ask an inquiry, breathe deeply and then go to sleep, hoping to get the answer in the morning.

Add a few drops to the gift of someone who is grieving to assist them in processing and manage better.

Incorporate into pillows for children (be cautious with boys prior to puberty-see the contradictions chapter) to encourage confidence and sleep

Mix rosemary with scent the room and clothes of your daughters to avoid sexual encounters that are premature to increase confidence and clarity.

Apply the cream behind your ears and on the neck's front to draw the opposite sexuality (adults)

Rub the frames of pictures of your loved ones to ensure their safety and to show your appreciation

Visualize and meditate on a successful using rosemary, lavender and rose oil, to gain confidence and self-assurance to pass tests or succeed at all things

Inhale whenever your vibration appears to be low.

Mix coconut oil and lavender essential oil. Use as a lubricant to perform sexual magic. Visualize the outcome of an orgasm. effective!

Apply lavender oil to ancestors and other altars to be able to communicate more effectively with spirits

Also I do not hold the title of a medical professional therefore, when discussing possible contraindications and safety issues, I'll refer readers to WebMD declarations below.Make your own choice regarding whether or not to utilize essential oils of lavender. It is not intended to dissuade you from using it, but rather let you know what the is the consensus of medical research on lavender.

According to WebMD, these are potential interactions with drugs.

Chloral Hydrate is a co-factor with LAVENDER.

Chloralhydrate can cause insomnia and the feeling of drowsiness. Lavender is thought to boost effect of the chloralhydrate. The combination of lavender and chloral hydrate could induce excessive somnolence.

Sedative drugs (Barbiturates) interact with LAVENDER

Lavender may cause sleepiness or Drowsiness. Sleep-inducing medications are referred to as sedatives. Combining lavender with sedative medicines could result in excessive sleepiness.

Some sedative drugs comprise amobarbital (Amytal) as well as butabarbital (Butisol) mephobarbital (Mebaral) pentobarbital (Nembutal) and phenobarbital (Luminal) and secobarbital (Seconal) as well as others.

Sedative medicines (CNS depressants) interact with LAVENDER

Lavender can cause sleepiness and Drowsiness. The medications that cause sleepiness are referred to as sedatives. The combination of lavender and sedative drugs could cause excessive sleepiness.

Certain sedative drugs include the clonazepam (Klonopin) and the lorazepam (Ativan) as well as Phenobarbital (Donnatal) and Zolpidem (Ambien) as well as others.

WebMD reports that according to WebMD,

Lavender is likely to be safe for the majority of adults when consumed in large quantities. It's POSSIBLY SAFE to take in the mouth or put on the body or inhaled in therapeutic amounts.

If taken orally when taken by mouth, lavender may cause headache, constipation, and an increase in appetite. If applied on the skin, lavender may cause irritation.

Special Precautions & Warns:

Children: Applying skin care products on the skin that contain lavender oil can be harmful for children who haven't yet reached puberty. Lavender oil is thought to have hormonal effects that can alter the normal hormones of the body of a boy. In some instances it has led to girls developing an abnormal growth of their breasts known as Gynecomastia. The dangers of these products being used by girls in their teens is not well-known.

Breast-feeding and pregnancies There isn't enough evidence-based information on the safety of lavender when you are breastfeeding or pregnant. Keep yourself safe and stay clear of use.

Operation: Lavender might slow down the central nervous system. If it is used in conjunction with anesthesia or other drugs used during and following surgery, it could reduce the nervous system to a great extent. Take lavender off at least 2 weeks prior to the scheduled surgery.

Chapter 14: Health And Wellness

Therapeutic Uses:

Since the beginning of time the world has been using essential oils for healing purposes.There are more than 200 references to ointments incense, and aromatics in both the ancient and modern testaments.In the oldest medical record "The Ebers Papyrus" over 800 remedies for herbal use and prescriptions are listed.

In the drug development prototypes that we have today, many were derived from plants oils.The medication aspirin came from the Birch tree.The rain forest serves as an important source of food for many treatment of various diseases, for instance 70% of the cancer drugs originate from it.

The problem is that drug companies alter plant oils in order that they are able to patent the oils in the form of"new" drugs "new" drug.They are not able to patent the oils of plants in their original state.The tragic fact is that a lot of people suffer from the adverse side effects of prescription medications that are currently the fourth largest causes of deaths across the United States.

Introduced back to Modern Medicine:

In the the 19th century and into the early 20th essential oils were introduced into the modern world of medicine.We have been learning every day about the therapeutic benefits from essential oil in our modern day society.

Researchers and doctors like Penoch, Valnet, Monuie and Gottefosse have made significant contributions as pioneers in our current understanding of the health advantages from essential oils.Dr. Gary Young a naturopath has committed his entire life to understanding the healing qualities of these oils.He is the creator of "Young Living Essential Oils."

Many essential oils have common properties that help us with various minor health concerns.Some of these properties are anesthetic, anti-fungal, anti-biotic, anti-septic, and anti-inflammatory.The majority of essential oils have at least two or more of these properties some have more.

Kit for Health and Wellbeing Kit:

Following is the list of the most essential oils you need to complete your wellness and health kit.

Clove Bud: sore throat and gums insect repellent burns, indigestion tension relieving headaches, acne and stress relief

Frankincense - cold and influenza asthma, anxiety as well as arthritis, bronchitis emotions, dry and flaky skin menstrual problems, scars, respiratory and dry skin

Oregano - allergies lice, gas, the bloating that can occur, mild fevers general cleaning solutions, digestion gum soreness and infections, burns, headaches and acne

Varicose veins – lemon mood enhancing Hard water stains general cleansing, warts take off the sticky labels, psoriasis cold sores, corns, athletes foot, minor wounds and cuts

Melaleuca (Tea Tree) is a remedy for respiratory illnesses such as bronchitis, chickenpox acne, fungal infection, bacterial, viral Cold sores cold and flu warts, corns, insect bites and head lice, dandruff and dry scalp

Peppermint - sinusitis and digestion issues nausea, decongestants, colic and fever. Scabies vertigo, asthma, and scabies

Rosemary is a great herb for mental clarity Stress and anxiety hair strengthening, arthritis and joint pain, the flu and cold, bad breath muscle pain and hair loss.

Lavender is a remedy for insomnia, earaches sunburn insects, headaches, depression and asthma as well as allergies, anxiety and acne

Chapter 15: Essential Oils For Mental Health

Life is now more difficult and stressful than ever before. There is no escape from the stresses of everyday life. You must build your mental capacity to face challenges by focusing on positive thoughts. Stress, anxiety depression, stress and failures keep appearing at all times of your life. Instead of becoming a subject to these negative feelings, you'll have to overcome them by focusing on your determination and positive thoughts. Essential oils can be used to boost your mood. The blends are able to make a positive atmosphere for you.

There are a variety of options in essential oils to use for your diffuser. You can make use of anything from citrus oil clary sage oil and basil oil, bergamot oil and frankincense oil. You can also use rose oils, geranium oil sandalwood oil wild orange oil Roman Chamomile oil, marjoram oil, lavender oil along with mandarin oils. All you have to do is use the diffuser in order for the best benefits.

When choosing essential oils to support your mental well-being You must choose the scent you prefer. It is not advisable to pick a scent that you don't like. If you do it will only cause negative consequences. You should use an oil that stimulates your positive feelings instead of choosing one that can produce negative ones. You want a stress-free serene, tranquil, and happy life.

Essential blend of recipes to improve mental health

1. For a relaxed and stress-free lifestyle

If your job is causing you lots of stress and your life isn't all that enjoyable You can make use of the essential oils blend in order to boost your mental state and help you stay relaxed in all situations. To make this blend, you'll require four drops of the sandalwood oil, four drops of ylang ylang oil two drops of lemon oil. The oils of sandalwood and ylang-ylang are believed to be effective in treating anxiety, and lemon oil is used to improve your mood. This blend is suitable to treat any type of depression and anxiety, including professional and personal.

To provide a safe and healthy atmosphere for all your family members it is possible to make a mixture of oils of the mandarin and rose as well as jasmine oils. It can create a healthier and serene environment at your home.

2. For cognitive performance

Many are thinking about different kinds of healthy drinks to boost the cognitive capabilities of their children. They are trying these strategies as early as they can. Students at universities and colleges also conduct research to find ways to boost their cognitive abilities and be more efficient. A lot of them don't realize that essential oils could aid in improving cognitive performance. You can make use of lavender oil and peppermint oils to achieve this goal. Lavender oil can be helpful in improving memory, and peppermint oil is beneficial to the cognitive capabilities of your. To make this blend, you'll need to mix a mixture consisting of 5 drops Lavender oil as well as 5 drops of Peppermint. It is possible to place this blend in your study space or at work to reap the advantages.

Chapter 16: Essential Oil Recipes for Relaxation and Stress Relievement

Stress has been shown to be among the most significant causes of ailments and even death in the most extreme cases. Our modern lifestyle puts us at risk of stress and that's why we have seen an upsurge in number of people seeking for solutions to stress. There are a variety of methods employed by various people to combat stress and the use of essential oils is one of them.

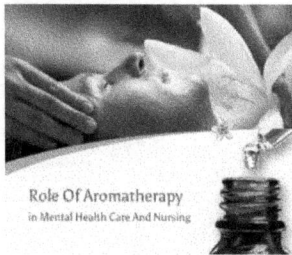

Role Of Aromatherapy
in Mental Health Care And Nursing

Essential oils can provide the feeling of calm and relaxation which is essential to be able to relax and unwind in our hectic life. Essential oils accomplish this through the use of aromatherapy.

There are many natural remedies you can utilize to get the happy and relaxing effect.You might be wondering if aromatherapy can aid in the reduction of stress. It stimulates the your endocrine and limbic systems. these are the organs that are responsible for hormones and emotional state. If this occurs, it triggers physical and emotional responses that is beneficial in this instance. A good example of this is when you are smelling Lavender essential oil. The tiny chemicals it contains activate your system, and it responds by calming the nervous system, resulting in relaxation of muscles.

There have been numerous studies that have been conducted to determine the connection with aromatherapy in stress relief and the results were favorable. It was discovered that patients who suffer from Alzheimer's disease were treated with lavender and lemon essential oils.

This diminished their levels of agitation. Depression sufferers took less antidepressants when they used lemon essential oil. Essential oils of ylang ylang were found to enhance endingorphin levels within the body. These are the hormones responsible for relieving pain and providing the feeling of healthy. Aromatherapy helps to reduce stress and relaxation.

The most potent essential oils that can help ease tension and stress include marjoram, lavender Melissa, geranium, cinnamon, vanilla, orange rose, neroli, Chamomile, ylang-ylang, and other essential oils.

Strategies to relieve stress through aromatherapy

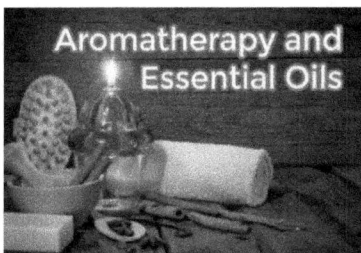

Aromatherapy and Essential Oils

I'm sure that you've heard many times to take self-care, but I'm here to remind you of this again. Self-care is vital to help your body combat stress. Many of us admit that we'd prefer to better take care of ourselves, but do not have the time. If you consider it, it's going cost you more the time you spend and also money neglect your health. Stop doing things that are too demanding. If you feel overwhelmed, you could take a break throughout the day to let yourself down.Doing this two times a every day for around five minutes is enough.You could increase the amount of time to around 15 minutes as your tolerance levels increase. If you are having trouble with this, then try the recipe for an aromatherapy inhaler.

Inhale your favorite aromatherapy scents at home

The convenience of having your own aromatherapy inhaler is fantastic because it's very lightweight. Therefore, you can carry it throughout the day because it's tiny and will be carried around in your purse, car, and you can utilize it at any time you require.

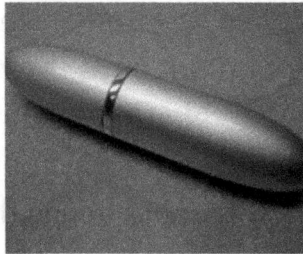

Ingredients

1 teaspoon of sea salt that is coarse.

10 drops in Bergamot essential oil.

4 drops of orange essential oil.

4 drops from Lavender Essential oil.

1 drop of chamomile or essential oil of Ylang ylang.

1 drop of Rose Essential oil of Geranium.

Glass bottles.

Procedure

Put the coarse sea salt inside a tiny and opaque glass bottle or dark plastic bottle.

Add the rest of the components to the mix.

Inhale the scent in three deep, slow breaths.

Relieve yourself for a few minutes and then inhale the scent for three breaths. Do this at least three times and you'll experience the most amazing aromatherapy to help relieve stress.

Mineral bath with a scent of Ylang Lemon and Ylang

Essential oils are wonderful in calming your mind and body. They are mildly relaxing and energizing and possess a fresh sweet scent.

Ingredients

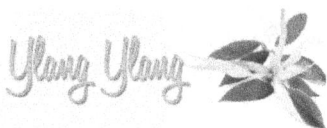

1 tablespoon baking soda.

2 teaspoons of sea salt.

1-1/2 tablespoons borax.

6 drops of essential lemon oils.

4 drops of ylang-ylang.

Procedure

Mix together baking soda, salt from the sea and borax.

Add the lemon and essential oils to the mix and mix it well.

Make a bath and put the mix in under the running water. Make sure that the salts dissolve completely and that the oils are evenly dispersed within the water. Add a few small drops Lavender to help create a healthy equilibrium.

Lavender, Chamomile and Tangerine blend

This blend is fantastic to relax and reduce stress. It helps the muscles, tissues and joints relax , and provide you a balanced energy.

Ingredients

3 drops of Tangerine.

3 drops of Lavender.

3 drops of Chamomile.

1 Ounce of carrier oil. (Choose any)

Procedure

Mix the essential oils mentioned above with the oil carrier.

Massage as desired.

The blend could also function as a bath oil.

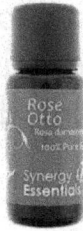

Rose Otto

The aroma of this is powerful and Aphrodisiac. It can benefit your body and mind. It is able to ease your stress and relax your anxiety. It can be enjoyed by taking a relaxing bath.

Ingredients

Bath water.

Three and a half tablespoons heavy cream.

3 drops of the essential Turkish Rose-Otto oil.

Procedure

Blend the cream heavy with Essential oil of Turkish Rose Otto.

Incorporate the mix into your bathwater.

Relax in your bath and soak in the water to relax and.

If you are looking for an aroma that is more sensual, you could add a few drops Jasmine and Sandalwood essential oils.

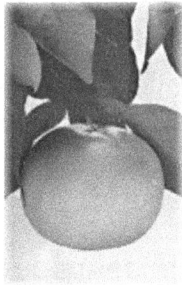

Tension taming recipes

This recipe for bath salts that smell aromatherapy can help ease tension. They accomplish this by stabilizing your nervous system, which can affect your mood as well. This recipe is very beneficial particularly for people with oily skin as it helps to cleanse the skin and decrease your production of oils, in addition to healing skin blemishes.

Ingredients

1 cup sea salt.

3 drops of Lavender Essential Oil.

6 drops in Bergamot Essential oil.

1/2 cup baking soda.

6 drops of Sweet Orange Essential oil.

4 drops from yellow, and 6 drops of food color. (This is an optional)

Procedure

Make use of a spoon made of metal to mix baking soda and salt. (A stainless steel spoon is suggested since a wooden spoon could be damaged from the absorption of vital oils).

Add a few drops of essential oils over the salts, and stir it until it's properly blended. Repeat the process for the food coloring.

Place the mixture in the jar of plastic or dark glass, and let it sit for 24 hours prior to using it.

One cup of salt is sufficient to make a bath. The recipe you've just created will be used up to three baths.

It is vital to know the fact that oranges sweet and Bergamot are not recommended to be consumed prior to being exposed to sunlight. This is because they can create photosensitivity and sunburn.

Recipe for Aromatherapy Bath Oil to relax

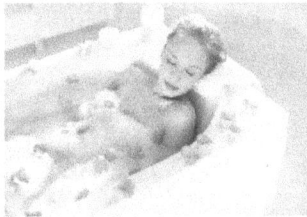

The recipe to make bath oils is extremely relaxing, and will make you feel calm and peaceful. All you have be able to do is breathe slow deep breaths and your worries will go away. The scent that is deep and calming of this bath oil is ideal for males. It can be used as a massage oil for your guy and help him calm down to the point that he may even sleep. Essential oil from Sandal Wood is one of the ingredients in this bath oil. It is essential for the healing of the skin. So if you suffer from skin issues like eczema and psoriasis, this bath oil is suitable for you. It also helps to reduce the appearance of eczema. it aids in slowing down the process of aging and reenergizes your skin.

Ingredients

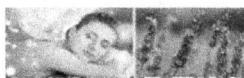

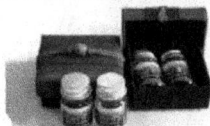

Lavender

12 drops from the Lavender Essential Oil.

4fl oz. equivalent to 125ml the carrier oil you like. Examples include almond and Jojoba oil.

30 drops from the Sandalwood Essential oil.

2 drops from Cedar Essential Oil for wood.

Procedure

Blend all ingredients inside a glass bottle (or dark glass). Place the bottle in an area that is cool and dark. (Keep the bottle away from your bathroom due to the humidity and warmth)

Add a tablespoon of the aromatic bath oil you created into the bath and let it run after you have used it.It is as easy as that, and you're looking forward to a relaxing bath to ease your anxiety.

Be wary of going for a cheap Sandalwood since it may not offer the same benefits as the original. It might be costly, but it's worth the money.

Aromatherapy bath oil to help you dream sweet dreams

This recipe for a bath is extremely relaxing and is particularly suitable for those suffering from insomnia. It will help you go to sleep. If you're experiencing an evening when it is difficult to fall asleep, then you don't have to be worried. Try this bath oil that will ease your stress and ease your muscles. Then, you'll be able to sleep peacefully in a state of calm as well. Additionally the essential oils aid in repairing your skin and lessen wrinkles. If you're not capable of taking a bath, or shower, you can massage your body and face with a bit of lavender oil, and you'll nevertheless enjoy its relaxing effect. It is recommended to do this prior to when you fall asleep so that you can get an uninterrupted sleep.

Did you think you could create the massage oils yourself? Yes, it's possible. While bath oils are essential but you might not have the time for the bath. But, if you own the massage oil, then you can utilize it for similar outcomes. Lavender is pleasant to the eyes It has a fantastic smell and has many healing properties so making Lavender oil for massage is wise choice.

Massage oil is excellent to ease pain,

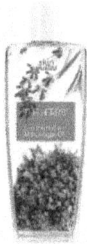

insomnia anxiety, stress and insomnia. If you can combine the incredible effects of Lavender along with its soft pressure, you're on the right track towards getting a full-on relaxation. If you're not able to get the full body massage, you could also try a foot massage. Massage oil can be massaged on your stomach and chest to aid in sleeping.

Ingredients

2 Drops from Clary Sage essential oil. Clary Sage essential oil.

12 drops from the Lavender Essential Oil.

3 drops of marjoram essential oil.

12 drops from or Orange Or Bergamot essential oils.

1 drop of essential oil Vetiver

1/4 cup of the carrier oil you like.

Procedure

1.Mix all ingredients in a glass bottle or dark glass. It is recommended to buy glasses or bottles that have an oil or lotion dispenser cup. This helps to prevent accidental spills.

2. You should wait at least 24 hours prior to using the massage to allow time for the "cure". The bottle must be kept in a dark, cool location and used within three months.

You can increase or decrease the amount of the ingredients, if you would like to get a huge quantity of massage oil.

The most important thing to keep in mind when selecting carriers oils, is the fact that you are able to modify them to meet the needs of your skin. It is recommended to select those that nourish and strengthen your skin.For instance, if you are using Jojoba or sweet almond oil, you could also include sea buckthorn oil or borage oil in case you are suffering from dry or mature skin. It's fine to play with various carrier oils to discover which works best for your skin. It's a great experience.

Chapter 17: What to Find The Best Essential Oils

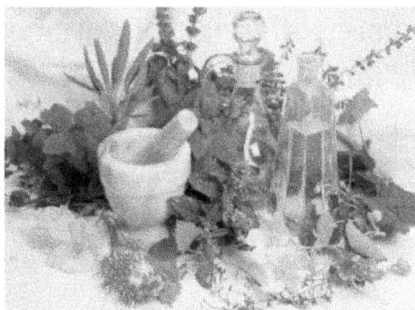

The choice of the best essential oil is a breeze. It's all about knowing your goal. If you're suffering from pain and aching, look for the essential oil that can relieve your sore muscles. If you're stressed then search for an essential oil that can provide an uplifting and relaxing effect. If you're feeling cramped and gassy, there's an oil that could ease the discomfort of indigestion.

Doesn't sound like a lot of work, does it?

The most difficult part is figuring out the things essential oils be used for and how to use it. Essential oils aren't only about choosing an oil bottle and spreading the contents over your desired region. It's not just about using an oil hoping for to see a quick miracle or "snap-of a-finger" kind of impact. You must know the most effective oil and the proper method to use it.

To reap the maximum benefits the benefits of essential oils and aromatherapy You must be thorough when conducting your study. There are a myriad of essential oils that perform the same function. For instance, chamomile and lavender are two examples. They provide both calming effects, however they smell slightly different from one other.By taking a look and doing your studies, you'll be in a position to narrow your search to just the essential oils that you require and desire.

Once you have identified your preferred oils However, there are additional factors you should consider when selecting the best essential oil. It's about:

*Cost

In general, premium essential oils are expensive. It could result from the time-consuming processing packaging, distribution and packaging companies must undergo to ensure the freshness of their product. However, you must remember that not all costly oil essentials are best.The cost could be an indication of the amount of concentrated or highly extracted the oils are. However, when the advertising sounds too appealing and believable, you should be more skeptical.

*Ingredients

As much as you can do your best to ensure that you look up the ingredient's labels. If you see something that is sounded like it's made of synthetic materials, you shouldn't purchase it. To make the most of essential oils it is recommended to choose organic oils. "Unsprayed" is an excellent term to discover in products as it indicates that no chemicals were spraying and splashed over plants that produce the.

*Purity

The more pure the oil, the greater the benefits you will reap. However, because processing is essential to preserve essential oils for longer, the majority of companies process them until the point that their quality is modified. If you're looking to purchase the essential oils, be sure you buy it from a reliable vendor or from people who specialize in this field. If you buy directly from them, you'll receive a legitimate product.

*Label

Along with ingredient scanning scans for expiry and distillation dates is also an essential. It is important to choose the product that's not just fresh , but also one that can be used for indefinitely. It won't be able to give you your money's worth if buy a product that's likely expire in just a few days, wouldn't it?

Brands are another thing you should think about. When you purchase an essential oil will give you greater peace of mind when you purchase an oil proven to be from a trusted source. Apart from the brand, make sure you check the label to see the origin, chemo kind and the country where the oil was extracted in.

Packaging

Packaging is one of the most important factors you must take into consideration when purchasing the bottle of essential oil. Bottles with amber colour and blue are excellent alternatives. Also, you should stay away from purchasing essential oils that include an empty dropper that is made of rubber inside the container. Rubber is known to break down over time and could affect the potency of your oil.

Instead of using a rubber dropper you can look for bottles that have been secured by orifice reduction. If you are worried about how you'll get a sufficient quantity of the product without dropping into a container, your ideal option is an glass pipette. It's also accurate, without the danger of altering the essential oil.

These factors aren't only important in determining the quality of the oil. They also provide an confidence that the product that you'll be using to treat your body will be secure and efficient. There are plenty of fake products available on the market, it is important to be cautious when making a decision to stay away from falling victim to fraud and scams. To ensure your security it is advisable to conduct an investigation to determine if the vendor you're dealing with offers genuine essential oils. In addition to the seller, you should be sure to do a google lookup on the company and reviews of other consumers on the product. If you know what others have to say, you can gain an idea of what to anticipate.

Chapter 18: Extraction Of Essential Oils

Essential oils are readily accessible for purchase at stores or markets. While some are sold in pure and concentrated form, some contain additives that make it less efficient. Commercially-marketed oils can also be costly in the long run.

But, the oils can extract at-home with the help of a home-based chemist. Once you have the proper equipment and you get the hang of it, it's fairly simple. Making your own oils can help you save money and will ensure that you receive the purest , most pure extracts.

There are many extraction methods that have evolved over decades from various locations. Some are more modern, and others are as ancient as time. Certain old techniques are also being developed and improved to increase their effectiveness.

Defluerage and Enfluerage

This is a traditional method that was employed primarily in perfumery. A large wooden frame is used along with a glass plate to form the equipment. The cold wax or another material similar to it is used for the base. Plant material is then put inside the apparatus and then placed on top of the glass sheets. Freshly cut flowers or plant parts are the most effective in this procedure. The plant parts are left to dry for around a day, before the extracts are removed with the help of Defluerage. The old material is taken away and replaced by new plants, flowers, and leaves. This is repeated in order to achieve the desired quantity of extracts but every time, the saturation levels can vary.

Expression

Expression, also known as cold pressing, is a different extraction method to extract essential oils. It is made by using hot water in order to soften leaves, flowers or other plant components. Then , a sponge is utilized to absorb this liquid, where the plant extracts are been dispersed. The oils and water are separated into different containers. In this process, it is crucial that the temperature does not exceed 120 degrees Fahrenheit. This procedure is quite slow when compared to other processes consequently it's not recommended.

Distillation

Raw materials get heated then cool to extract the substances during this process. The distillation can be three different types:

1)Water distillation

2)Direct steam distillation

3.) Steam distillation and water

Raw materials get then steamed in sills. The oils are released out of them by heating. They also evaporate in the steam that is later stored. The steam is then condensed, and the oil is separated.

These steps will assist you complete a low-cost distillation process at your home.

Distillation at Home

Materials:

Pressure cooker

Stove

Plant materials

Copper tube

Glass containers

Glass tub

Method:

1)First take all the raw materials in the pressure cooker. After that, place it on top of a stove. Fill it to the point that less than an inch is left at an upper part of your cooker.

2)Then add boiling drinking water on the materials, and close the cooker completely. Then turn off the gas. The temperature should rise to around 210 degrees F.

3.) Make a tub and fill it up with cold water. Put it in the vicinity of your cooker.

4)Connect the copper tube with the cooker, and then run it through the cold water tub.

5)The opposite end of the tube must be placed into the glass jar.

6.) It is expected that the oils expand when they are in cold water and are stored in the container.

7) Then , use an unwashed fabric such as cheesecloth to remove the oils. This is the final product.

It's fairly cheap to perform the distillation at your home. Once you've mastered it, it can become an enjoyable pastime. It is possible to get a high-quality extract once you've become more proficient at it. The following tips can ensure you have a high quality extract:

Use high quality of raw ingredients. Make sure that they are of the quality of the essential oil is the top of the line. The healthy plants that are that are harvested at the correct moment will yield the finest extract. It is equally crucial to select the right parts of the plant. Plants grown in the local area are the best since they don't contain the same amount of insecticides and other potentially harmful components.

Remove any contaminants or dirt from the plant material prior to distilling them. In the event that you don't, your extract could be affected.

It is also recommended to dry your plant materials before you use them since it will provide greater extract for each batch.

Different plants have different ideal times for carrying the distillation process, so be aware of that also.

Keep the oils out of sunlight since they could alter and degrade. A dark and cool place is ideal.

Glass bottles with dark colors are suitable to store essential oils. They can last for as long as two years in most cases.

Do not use any plastic material for your device. Aluminium, copper, as well as stainless steel make the ideal material for your components.

Chapter 19: Aromatherapy Health Benefits of Aromatherapy

Do you realize that your brain are able to discern 10,000 distinct scents? Simply take a whiff and you'll detect an distinct scent. Go outside and sniff the air. It's something else, isn't it? Everyone enjoys the scent of flowers or the aroma of freshly-baked apple tart. There's the total opposite - the sour and unpleasant smell of exhaust emissions. You don't want to be waking up in a room laden with unwelcome smells, right? The body is able to distinguish between a pleasant and a bad smell for an reason. The body can tell the scent that is harmful and which one is good.This instinctual sense also serves to protect as well as an ability to differentiate between two scents.

You might have noticed that smells can affect your mood also. Smell is among of the strongest senses that a human being has. It is important to note that aromatherapy isn't just about pleasing scents. There are many health benefits , including the following:

Feeling of relaxation, and the immediate release of tension

The sense of having an emotional well-balanced

An improved mood and feeling of wellbeing

*Relief from anxiety

*Boosting the immune system

There are numerous situations in which aromatherapy can make a difference. Many people enjoy aromatherapy due to the fact that it is a natural remedy that enhances the health. It's not an alternative to medical treatments as claimed by certain. If someone claims that aromatherapy can heal the symptoms of an illness, it may not be true. However, essential oils are extremely effective in relieving pain. I'll provide the essential oils as well as some methods to give you that revitalizing aroma you've sought for.

It is essential to conduct research prior to trying something. Essential oils aren't going to harm you in any way , except the case of applying the concentrated oil of lemon on your skin, and this might not be a wise choice. It's not going to hurt your skin, but it could increase the chance of suffering from sunburn.

Essential oils: What are you do with these oils?

Blending various oils to create synergy. Blending different oils it increases the potency of each and resulting in more effective outcomes. There are many levels of strength. It is possible to achieve synergy using various recipes, but you must adhere to precisely the instructions. Certain oils require to mature before they are suitable for use as the form of a "carrier oil".

Diluting them

Once you've selected your essential oil, you can include your preferred cosmetic or health ingredient to complement the aroma of the oil. Making essential oils more diluted is simple and you can mix them in with bath oils shower gels, lotions, shower and body/massage lotions.

Essential oils can be used in a variety of ways:

Massage

To massage, you may use five drops that are your base oils.

For Inhalation

Simply drop the 2 drops you want of your preferred essential oil into boiling water or onto an absorbent tissue to inhale.

While taking a Bath

It is as simple as placing 7-10 drops into the tub, which is filled with warm water.

Utilizing It in the Sauna

Simply add 2 drops to the hot water of a pot and drink it up.

Use It for Face-lifts

Simply add 3-4 drops of your preferred blend in the product base.

Foot Bath

Relieve exhausted feet by putting 10-drops of your favourite blend in the bowl of warm water.

Use It To Clean Your Face Pack and Sauna

Simply put 12 drops of water into a bowl of water.

Utilize As A Cleanser

20 drops in four one ounces of base product are enough to cleanse your body thoroughly.

Apply It To Your Body

Simply add 8-15 drops to the base product and then enjoy the fragrance.

Upper Body Rub

10-20 drops per 2 2 oz. of carrier oil, rub it lightly all over your chest.

Scent Your Clothes

Make use of it to add scent to the washing machine.

Simply add 10-20 drops per load to get your clothes scented.

Use a scent for your vacuum cleaner:

Simply add 5-10 drops into your cleaning machine, and then give your carpet a scent and floors.

Parfum Your Christmas Tree

Simply add 10-15 drops into your tree to give fragrance to your space.

Carrier Oils are usually used in conjunction in conjunction with Essential Oils

Essential oils tend to diminish very fast.With the loss of their properties, their healing properties are also diminished. To preserve all the healing and goodness essential oils are usually blended along with various oils. The most frequently used oil carrier is:

*Almond Oil

*Jojoba Oil

*Olive Oil

* Grapeseed Oil

*Avocado Oil

*Coconut Oil

Strategies for Effectively Using Essential oils

Essential oils are now gaining popularity and popular among the general public to use in their daily lives. What we need to be aware of is the fact that they are a natural oil extracted by distilling the plant or another sources from which it is extracted, and possesses its distinctive fragrance".In the sense that it is the essential ingredient of plants.

The essential oils can be used in a myriad of ways! They are used for everything from healing your body to cleaning your home. Essential oils are 100% organic and can be used for a variety of purposes. It is due to this nature that they are extremely appealing. If you are seeking an organic, chemical free method to live their life essential oils are crucial to achieve the desired goal.

Utilizing essential oils at home is much simpler than you could ever imagine. Here's an inventory of the most well-known applications of essential oils and how to utilize the oils in a way that will make the most of them.

Natural Carpet Deodorizer

To create a natural Carpet deodorizer all that you have to do is mix baking soda and 7 to 6-7 drops of essential oils. For instance the oils of lavender or orange can be a good option for this. Mix baking soda and oils thoroughly. Put them in shaker. Sprinkle it on your carpet and leave at least 10 minutes. The baking soda will soak up the unpleasant smells while the oils will leave the carpet clean and clean. Then, you can vacuum your carpet just like normal.

Air Freshener Plug-In Refill

The aroma of essential oils is so powerful that they are the top air fresheners in your home. For instance, put the drops of your preferred essential oil on a tiny piece of fabric and put it into the dryer. The dryer's heat will trigger the scent and will make your clothes and whole space smell amazing!

If you're aware that air freshener plug-in containers are made from glass, then you shouldn't throw them out of the window from now on. This is because you are able to refill them and reuse them with essential oils that are great.

It's not difficult to do. Simply use a sharp knife to cut the freshener. Fill the glass container to half full using the essence oil you believe is your preferred. The rest of the container should be filled with water that has been filtered. Shake it vigorously until the water and oil are evenly mixed. Replace the wick, and then plug it in the same way as you would normally. The use of essential oils to freshen the air does not only help you save money, but also makes it far healthier.Also it's an organic alternative to the components of a plug-in air purifier.

The most popular oils you can use to accomplish this are citrus, peppermint and cinnamon. For a more interesting smell it is possible to mix several oils. For example, mix cinnamon with orange as well as vanilla with orange. This can make it more adaptable.

Homemade Fabric Freshener

It's not difficult to make a wonderful home-made fabric refresher. This is how you can create a fabric freshener at your own home. Take a good-sized spray bottle. Make 1 tablespoon of baking soda 2 cups of water, and 10-drops of essential oil. Mix the essential oil with baking soda in a dish using an fork. Put the mixture in the spray bottle and add water. Shake the mix before you use it again. Include essential oils individually depending on your preference or mix two or three to create a stronger smell.

Conclusion

I hope that this book will serve you effectively. There's plenty of information online concerning oil essentials and use. There are forums on the internet which can further stimulate your curiosity. I've done my best to help you get startedand I'm sure these recipes will help you enhance your health.

www.ingramcontent.com/pod-product-compliance
Lightning Source LLC
Chambersburg PA
CBHW060333030426
42336CB00011B/1319